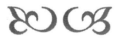

Celebrating Holidays
~Gluten-Free~

An Invaluable Guide to Celebrating
Holidays Gluten-Free Year-Round

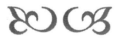

Karen E. Ruckman

authorHOUSE®

AuthorHouse™
1663 Liberty Drive
Bloomington, IN 47403
www.authorhouse.com
Phone: 1-800-839-8640

First published by AuthorHouse 8/9/2010

ISBN: 978-1-4520-1643-6 (sc)
ISBN: 978-1-4520-1644-3 (e)

Printed in the United States of America
Bloomington, Indiana

This book is printed on acid-free paper.

This book is dedicated to my beautiful granddaughter, Abigail Maria. May she always enjoy celebrating holidays as much as her Grammy.

℘ INTRODUCTION ℭ

Celebrating Holidays ~Gluten-Free~ has been an ongoing collaboration of mine since my children were little. I started a scrapbook of family recipes and historical information on holidays when my firstborn was two. As the years have gone by, I have revamped my favorite recipes to be gluten free. Even though I haven't been diagnosed with celiac disease, I do have fibromyalgia, arthritis and hypothyroidism and find eating gluten free foods make me feel better. In searching for gluten free cookbooks, I didn't find any that centered solely on celebrating holidays, thus, my reason for putting this cookbook together.

Eating gluten free today has become much easier with all the manufacturers that now produce gluten free foods and the stores that carry them. In converting my recipes, I found that for some it was only necessary to use a gluten free brand of the product called for. Therefore, in my recipes you will find that I have mentioned brand names to help you find a product that is gluten free. Now, you may have a favorite brand name that I have not mentioned, that's ok; use your brand it should work fine.

A few things I want to point out:
1. *If you cannot tolerate dairy, feel free to use dairy free substitutions.*
2. *All seasonings even though not mentioned are McCormick Brand.*
3. *If you have a favorite gluten free recipe for a prepared item mentioned by all means use it.*
4. *I have used Bob's Red Mill All Purpose Gluten Free Flour throughout the book, but if you have a favorite combination of gluten free flours you should try them in the recipe. It is cheaper to make up your own batch of gluten free flour than to buy readymade. One of my favorites is 3 cups of brown and/or white rice flour, 1 cup of potato flour, ½ cup of tapioca flour and 1 tablespoon of xanthan gum.*

This book is for anyone who wants to live well without gluten. It is amazing how good the recipes are and how easy they are to make.

I hope this cookbook inspires you to be creative and to enjoy your holidays living your best, most healthful life.

Karen E. Ruckman

❦ CONTENTS ❧

❧ JANUARY ☙

Overall Theme: Snow – Snowman
Colors: Blue, Silver, and White

"AULD LANG SYNE"
By Robert Burns

Should auld acquaintance be forgot and never brought to mind?
Should auld acquaintance be forgot and days of auld lang syne?

For auld lang syne, my dear, for auld lang syne,
we'll take a cup o' kindness yet for auld lang syne.

And here's my hand my trusty frien', and gie's a hand o' thine;
we'll take a right gude-willi waught for days of auld lang syne.

For auld lang syne, my dear, for auld lang syne,
we'll take a cup o' kindness yet for auld lang syne.

New Year's Day

Centerpiece - Resolution Basket

On New Year's Day ask family members to write down their hopes and resolutions for the year ahead. Put them into envelopes and seal them. Then next year, have fun reading the notes to see if they've come true.

Breakfast: New Year's Fritters

2 c milk
1/2 c butter
3 eggs
1/2 c Dominos sugar
1 t salt
2 c Sun Maid raisins
2 envelopes of Fleischmann's dry yeast
4 to 5 c Bob's Red Mill all purpose flour

Scald milk; cool to lukewarm and add remaining ingredients and mix well. Let rise until double in bulk. Drop into hot, deep fat by tablespoonfuls and fry until brown. Serves 8.

Dinner: Hoppin' John
to bring wealth (pork for rutting forward)

1 lb dried black eyed peas
1/2 lb Hormel salt pork, cubed
1/2 lb cooked Hormel ham, cubed
1 large onion, chopped
3 garlic cloves, minced
1/4 t crushed red pepper
pepper to taste
3 c cooked rice

Rinse peas and pick over, removing any small stones or foreign particles. Cover with cold water in a large pot, bring to a boil for a minute, and remove from heat cover and let sit for one hour. In a large skillet, sauté the salt pork to render fat, add onion and garlic and cook until onion is soft, about 5-6 minutes. Add the onion mixture and seasonings to the pot with the peas. Add enough water to cover the ingredients and bring to a simmer. Cover and cook for about 1- 1 1/2 hours or until black-eyed peas are tender but not mushy. Season with salt and pepper to taste. Serve over hot cooked rice. Serves 8-10.

Martin Luther King's Birthday

Martin Luther King, Jr. fought for freedom and equality for everyone. He preached and lived nonviolence, and won the Nobel Peace Prize. His favorite food was pecan pie. Serve a slice with Chocolate Swizzle Nog

Pecan Pie

1 1/2 c chopped pecans
3/4 c Dominos packed brown sugar
1/2 c Bob's Red Mill All Purpose Flour
1/4 c softened butter
3/4 c milk
3/4 c Karo's light corn syrup
1 1/2 t vanilla
4 eggs

Preheat oven to 350° F. Spray a 9 inch pie plate with vegetable spray. Sprinkle pecans in bottom of pie plate. Combine all remaining ingredients with a fork. This batter will be lumpy. Pour over pecans. Bake 45-50 minutes or until knife inserted in middle comes out clean. Let stand 15 minutes. Serve plain or with ice cream.

Chocolate Swizzle Nog

1 c Carnation's instant dry milk
1/3 c hot water
1/2 c Dominos sugar
1 T melted butter

Mix ingredients in blender until smooth. Pour into a medium-sized saucepan and combine **2 c milk** and **2 T Hershey's unsweetened cocoa powder**. Heat through, stirring constantly. Remove from heat. Stir in **½ t vanilla or peppermint extract**. Serve warm in mugs; top with **Cool Whip**. Store covered in refrigerator. Serves 4.

℘ FEBRUARY ℀

Overall Theme: Hearts
Colors: Red, White, and Blue

Super Bowl Sunday

Begin with an invitation. Photocopy part of the sports page from the newspaper or a sports magazine. Write your party details in one of the columns. Ask guests to dress in their team colors.

Create a centerpiece. Arrange a bunch of pennants in a foam ball and place the ball inside a football helmet. Add crushed soda cans and trading cards to your centerpiece.

For a buffet table covering, use football T-shirts, jerseys, jackets or sweatshirts. Decorate your table with green felt or Astroturf and use white tape as yard lines. Use wooden dowels for goal posts.

Decorate the room with your favorite team colors using crepe paper streamers and football Mylar balloons. Suspend football posters and pennants in your party room. You can create team pennants from colored card stock and attach to wooden sticks. Hang a Football piñata and let the kids break it.

Super Bowl Menu

Super Bowl Chili

1-16 oz can chopped tomatoes, do not drain
2-15 oz cans dark red kidney beans, not drained
1 lb ground beef
1 small red pepper (chopped)
1 1/2 c water
1 clove garlic
1/8 t pepper
1 t ground cumin
1 onion, chopped
1 T chili powder
2 T Dominos sugar
1 T dried oregano

Brown ground beef in large saucepan, drain grease. Add water and seasonings. Let simmer approx. 10 minutes. Remove mixture to large pot. Add tomatoes, kidney beans, and pepper. Bring to a boil; reduce heat, and simmer approx. one half-hour. Make a day ahead and reheat during the second quarter so it will be ready for half time. Top heated chili with shredded cheddar cheese and green onions. Serves: 8-10

Chicken Salad

4 1/2 c diced cooked chicken
1 1/2 c diced apples
3/4 c halved green grapes
6 T Trader Joe's sweet pickle relish
6 T Hellman's mayonnaise
6 T Wish Bone ranch salad dressing
1/2 t salt

In a large bowl, combine the chicken, apples and grapes. In a small bowl, combine the pickle relish, mayonnaise, ranch dressing, and salt. Pour over chicken mixture and toss to coat. Serve in a **lettuce**-lined bowl. Serves: 18

Popcorn

4 qt Jiffy Pop popped corn
12 oz Good Sense peanuts
2 c shredded Kraft cheddar cheese
1/4 c melted butter
2 t each lemon pepper, cumin, chili powder, paprika

Combine popcorn, peanuts, and cheese in a large bowl. Set aside. Add spices to melted butter one at a time, stirring constantly. Pour over popcorn and toss to coat. Serves 6.

Nachos

1 lb ground beef
1 small onion, diced
salt and pepper to taste
1-16 oz can Ortega refried beans
1-14.5 oz pkg Tostitos unflavored tortilla chip
2-8 oz pkgs shredded Kraft Cheddar & Monterey Jack cheese

In a large frying pan, brown ground beef with onion, salt and pepper over medium heat. Break the meat into very small pieces while it is cooking. After the meat is thoroughly cooked, drain off the grease.

Arrange chips on a microwavable platter. Spread beans over the chips. Layer with 1/2 of the cheese, the ground beef mixture, and then remaining cheese. Microwave on medium high until cheese has melted. Serve with Breakstone's regular sour cream and Chi-Chi's salsa. Makes 6 servings.

Build Your Own-Sundae-Buffet

Use different flavors of ice cream and lots of different toppings of your choice.

Valentine's Day

St. Valentine's Day originated from several events and customs. It is named after St. Valentine, who was a Christian priest. The origins of Valentine's Day can be traced back to Pagan times.

In ancient Rome, February 14th was a day honoring Juno, the Goddess of women and marriage and Queen of the Roman Gods and Goddesses. The following day, February 15th, began the Feast of Lupercalia, a festival of love honoring Juno. Love lotteries were an important component of the celebration, which took place on the eve of the festival. The names of girls were written on slips of paper and placed into jars. Young men would draw a girl's name from the jar, making these two partners for the duration of the festival. So even though they weren't yet called by the name, these early Romans were in fact the first Valentines. Of course, the early Christians frowned on such erotic goings-ons.

Saint Valentine or Valentinus, who had been martyred on February 14th 269 A.D, proved a convenient symbol around which to fashion the toning down nature of Lupercalia from eroticism to romance. While evidence suggests the saint was himself a chaste man, legend has it he defied Emperor Claudius II by secretly marrying count- less couples, a practice the emperor had banned believing that marriage weakened his army. Eventually Claudius caught on and the good saint was condemned and beaten to death.

Another legend has it that Valentinus had befriended his jailer's daughter during his imprisonment. He left her a farewell letter signed "From Your Valentine".

In 496 AD, Pope Gelasius set aside February 14 to honor St. Valentine, who became the patron saint of lovers and gradually, February 14 became a day for exchanging love messages and simple gifts. The practice of lottery drawings to select Valentines persisted well into the eighteenth century, but a gradual shift took place in which the gift giving became the sole responsibility of the man. This marked the beginning of the end and the practice eventually disappeared and individuals were at last free to select their own Valentines.

Manufactured Valentine cards didn't appear until the end of the eighteenth century. The Victorians took the cards to elaborate lengths, trimming them with lace, silks and satins and embellishing them with special details like feathers, flowers, gold leaf, hand painted details and even sweetly perfumed sachets. Until the mid-1800's, the cost of sending mail was beyond the means of the average person, and the recipient, not the sender was expected to pay the cost of mailing.

It wasn't until the advent of the penny post that the modern custom of sending Valentine's cards really gained critical mass. Today, Valentine's Day is the second most popular occasion for sending greeting cards, only surpassed by Christmas.

Tips for your Valentine's Day Party

Serve simple cookies and punch on doily lined plates. Set up a table for the kids to make homemade Valentine's while they are at the party. You could even set up another table for everyone to decorate their own sugar cookies! Make sure you keep everything simple.

Rosemary Valentine Wreath
Give this dainty, heart-shaped decoration to your Valentine or lovingly decorate your home.

Heavy-gauge wire
Wire cutters
Slender sprays of rosemary
Florists silver wire
4 Wheat stalks
Scissors
Dried herbs/flowers such as rosebuds, lady's mantle, Queen Anne's lace and strawflower
Satin ribbon, 1/2 inch wide

Although, traditionally red roses and rosebuds signify true love, include some yellow roses and cream flowers to lighten the design a little and to give it variety.

The rosemary symbolizes love, fidelity and remembrance. The wheat symbolizes riches, prosperity and friendliness. A single red rose symbolizes everlasting love. Yellow roses symbolize joy. Pink roses symbolize perfect happiness.

Twist the wire into a circle. Then, by pinching it at the base and the top, make it into a heart shape. You can make it any size you want, but the one I made measures 8 inches in length. Cut short sprays of rosemary and bind two or three together on the frame with silver wire. Place together two wheat stalks. Cut two more stalks into several short lengths and fasten these to the top of the two long stalks. They will form the top of the decoration. Bind short sprays of rosemary and the dried flowers along the length of the stalk, placing the rosebuds so that they face in opposite directions. Tie the ribbon close to the top of the stalks so that it conceals the first stem binding. Fasten the stalk to the top and base of the heart and tuck in small flower sprays to conceal the wires. Wire a single red rose to the inside center of the heart. The rosemary will gradually dry on the decoration if it is hung in a warm, dry atmosphere. Then it will become a lasting token. Note: The decorated wheat stalks run vertically up and down in the center of the wreath.

Favorites for Sweetest Day Gifting

Heart Shaped Pins
These make nice presents for Parents, Grandparents, Teachers, and Friends

1 c flour
1 c warm water
2 t cream of tartar
1 t oil
1 c salt
Red Food Coloring

Mix together the flour, water, cream of tartar, oil, and salt. Stir over medium heat until smooth, adding food coloring at the end. Remove from the pan. When cool enough to handle, knead until well blended. Shape into hearts and press pins into the backs of the hearts.

Valentine Hearts Pin

Take one **red or pink pipe cleaner** and cut in half. Twist ends together. Shape to make a heart. Add a **safety pin**. Give to a friend.

Make Your Own Valentine Paper

On the table, place **white paper** and **various heart-shaped cookie cutters**. Pour **red and pink paint** in shallow pans - **Styrofoam trays** work as well. Print hearts on white paper using the cookie cutters as a tool.

Variation: Print on tissue paper. Makes great wrapping paper

Stained Glass Heart

Place **red, pink, and white crayon shavings** between two pieces of **waxed paper** or in waxed paper sandwich bag. Cover with **newspaper**. Adult presses with warm **iron** to melt crayon chips. Allow to cool. Fold **construction paper** in half to make card. Cut heart shape from front of card. Tape "stained glass" behind the heart-shaped hole.

Variation: Cut "stained glass" into heart shape. Attach string to create mobile.

Herbal Potpourri Valentines

2 oz sweet woodruff
1 oz each red rose petals and red clover tops
3 oz rose hips
3 vanilla beans, sliced
1 oz orris root, cut
30 drops essential oil of choice
muslin, lace, ribbon

Cut muslin hearts and sew together sachets, leaving an opening for the herbs. Tuck some of the potpourri mixture into each sachet; close up opening and trim with lace and a ribbon for hanging.

The RoMANtic Valentines Worth Sending

If you are going to celebrate Valentine's Day, I suggest you do it with a little forethought. Buy your card now and mail it out to Loveland, Colorado for extra special treatment. Your card will be postmarked LOVEland, Colorado and it will also be hand-stamped with a unique four line poem.

The Loveland Chamber of Commerce organizes this yearly romance project with cards going to all 50 states and over 100 foreign countries.

It's simple. Just enclose your pre-addressed, pre-stamped Valentine's card in a larger envelope and mail to:

Postmaster, Attn: Valentines, Loveland CO 80537.

Here are some more "romantic" cities.

Kissimmee, Florida 32741
Valentine, Texas 79854
Valentine, Nebraska 69201
Loving, New Mexico 88256
Bridal Veil, Oregon 97010
Romance, Arkansas 72136

The Chocolate Theory

Chocolate Balls
These look great wrapped up in Plastic Wrap then tied with a Red ribbon

Mix ingredients in blender until smooth:
1 c Carnations instant dry milk
1/3 c hot water
1/2 c Dominos sugar
1 T melted butter

Next melt 3 c of **Hershey's semi-sweet or white chocolate chips**; remove from heat. Stir in blender ingredients. Chill 3 hours or until firm. Shape into 1 - inch (2.5cm) balls; place on wax paper-lined trays. Chill until firm.

Roll in finely chopped **Good Sense nuts** and **Hershey's cocoa powder**, or dip into melted **chocolate chips** of a different color. Chill and enjoy. Makes 5 dozen.

Chocolate Butter

Stir **1 stick of softened butter**; cut into pieces and **¼ cup melted Hershey's semi-sweet chocolate chips** together by hand. Transfer to covered container, refrigerate or freeze until ready to use. Serve with biscuits, pound cake, croissants, muffins or waffles.

Chewy Chocolates

1/2 lb soft caramels
2 T heavy cream
1 c Good Sense pecan halves
4 squares semi-sweet Hershey's chocolate, melted and cooled

Heat caramels with cream in a saucepan over very low heat, stirring constantly. Cool 10 minutes. Set pecans on lightly buttered baking sheets in clusters of 3. Spoon caramel mixture over nuts, leaving outer ends of nuts showing. Let stand to set, about 30 minutes. Spread melted chocolate over caramel mixture. Makes 2 dozen.

Candy Grams

I "chews" you for my Valentine (Trident stick of gum)
This may be "corny", but be my Valentine (candy corn)
"Mint" to ask you to be mine (mint)
A "kiss" for you if you'll be mine (Hershey's kiss)
Don't burst my "bubble" - Be mine (bubble gum)
I'm no "sucker" - I want you for my Valentine (lollipop)

Romantic Valentine's Day Dessert

Sweetheart Cake

2 envelopes unflavored gelatin
1/4 c cold water
1/2 c Dominos sugar
1/2 c crushed Dole pineapple w/juice
2 T ReaLemon juice
1/4 c maraschino cherry juice
2-3oz pkgs Philadelphia regular cream cheese, softened
12 cherries (quartered)
3 drops Cake Mate red food coloring
1-12 oz container of Cool Whip

Soften gelatin in cold water and set aside. In a saucepan, boil sugar and pineapple juice. Remove from heat and add gelatin, lemon juice and cherry juice. Cool to lukewarm. Whisk in cream cheese until blended. Stir in cherries and food coloring. Chill until slightly thickened then fold in whipped topping. Pour into a 9 x 13 baking dish, and refrigerate. Serves: 8

President's Day

For Breakfast prepare:

3 small Indian Hoecakes (a cake of cornmeal, water, and salt baked) w/tea

Dinner: Lincoln Log

1-8-oz pkg Philadelphia regular cream cheese, softened
1-4 oz c Kraft cheddar cheese, shredded
1/2 c diced red onion
1T Lea & Perrins Worcestershire sauce
1 t celery seed
1/2 c chopped Good Sense walnuts
2-3 fresh rosemary or parsley sprigs
Assorted Mary's Gone Crackers

In a mixing bowl, combine first 5 ingredients; beat until fluffy. Cover and refrigerate for at least 2 hours. Shape into a 7-in. x 1-1/2-in. log; roll in walnuts. Insert rosemary or parsley sprigs for branches. Serve with crackers. Makes 2 cups.

Washington Apple Pizza

1/2 c Philadelphia regular cream cheese
2 T minced onion
1/2 t dried dill weed
16-oz pre-cooked Ener-G Foods pizza crust
2 c Golden Delicious apples, cored and thinly sliced
1 c thinly sliced sweet red pepper
3/4 cup shredded part-skim Kraft mozzarella cheese

Combine cream cheese, onion and dill; mix well. Spread on pizza crust. Layer apples, and peppers on cheese mixture. Sprinkle with mozzarella cheese on top. Bake at 450° F about 7 minutes or until mozzarella cheese is thoroughly heated. Serves 6 to 8.

Little Logs

Bake a **white GF cake mix** in paper baking cups as directed on package or use the recipe that follows. Remove papers after cake cools.

White Cake

2 c Bob's Red Mill all-purpose flour
2 t xanthan gum
1 1/2 c Domino's sugar
1 t salt
3 1/2 t Calumet baking powder
1/2 c Crisco shortening
1 c milk
1 t vanilla
3 eggs

Heat oven to 350° F. Grease and flour paper liners for muffin tins. Measure all ingredients into a large bowl. Blend 1/2 minute on low speed, scraping bowl constantly. Beat 3 minutes on high speed, scraping bowl occasionally. Pour into muffin tins. Bake 15-20 minutes for cupcakes or until wooden pick inserted in center comes out clean. Cool.

Put two cupcakes together end to end with **Pillsbury chocolate fudge frosting** to form logs. Frost sides, leaving ends of logs (tops of cupcakes) unfrosted. With tines of fork, make lines in frosting to resemble bark. Decorate each log with a hatchet cut from construction paper.

Fastnacht Day

Fastnacht Day is a special Pennsylvania Dutch tradition that falls on Shrove Tuesday (the day before Ash Wednesday).

The tradition is to eat the very best before the Lenten fast. Therefore, Fastnachts. The lard called for may be replaced with vegetable oil.

The "proper" Pennsylvania Dutch way to eat a Fastnacht is to slice through center (as you would a bagel) and spread with molasses, King Syrup or "Turkey Brand" syrup. Some prefer to also spread with butter first.

FASTNACHTS: MAKES 2-1/2 DOZEN

2 c milk, scalded and cooled to lukewarm
3/4 c Dominos sugar
1/3 c Crisco or vegetable oil
1 t salt
1 pkg Fleischmann's dry yeast, dissolved in 1/2 c lukewarm water
2 eggs, beaten
Bob's Red Mill all-purpose flour to stiffen, about 3 pounds
1 pinch nutmeg

Mix together all ingredients except flour. Gradually add flour, stirring well, using spoon until thick. Then use hands and start kneading, gradually adding more flour until no longer sticky. Cover with wet cloth and let rise in warm place for about 4 hours.

Roll dough on floured board to 1/2 to 3/4-inch thickness. Cut into rectangles about 2-1/2 x 3-1/2 inches. Make hole in center. Place on floured board and let rise about 1 hour.

Deep fry in lard or vegetable oil at 360° F until golden brown. Flip to other side and brown. Drain on paper towels. (Recipe can easily be doubled).

Mix Dominos powered sugar with a bit of nutmeg. Dust with powdered sugar while still warm.

Mardi Gras Madness

For those not living in the South, February 27 is Mardi Gras. This day marks the end of a season of parties, merriment and celebrations before the onset of lent.

Mardi Gras began in Mobile, Alabama and is still celebrated there in grand style today. -- Visitors to Mobile can view dazzling Mardi-Gras costumes as well as other Fat Tuesday historical memorabilia, year round, at the Museum of Mobile located at 355 Government Street (334-208-7569).

Mardi Gras is also celebrated in New Orleans, of course, but you can find parades and festivities in most of the towns that dot the gulf coast in Louisiana, Mississippi and Alabama, Families will especially find some the smaller celebrations more appealing than that of New Orleans.

Mardi Gras is the height of the Southern Social season. It's a wild, raucous party for a month or more leading up to the big day. It is accompanied by endless rounds of formal balls, preceded over by elaborately costumed courts. Each ball is sponsored by a "Krewe" which also foots the bill for a parade or float in a larger parade, depending on the size and budget of the krewe.

The word "krewe" was supposedly chosen to give an "Old English" feel the clubs. Can I go to a ball you ask? Sorry Cinderella, Mardi-Gras balls are private affairs and by invitation only. However, you could get lucky and meet someone in the krewe who might just invite you. Your chances are increased significantly depending upon your sex. Many balls follow the 5-1 ratio tradition. In other words, if it's a men's krewe, each male member invites five women to the ball. The reverse is true if it is a women's krewe. Those Southerners know how to party! Also, keep in mind that, just like other Mardi-Gras events, there are plenty of balls outside of New Orleans.

A Mardi Gras Parade is different than other parades because they're interactive and you get things. Masses of screeching parade enthusiasts, arms outstretched like beggars clamoring for a last meal, beseech Krewe members to throw barrels of trinkets -- colorful plastic beads and imprinted aluminum doubloons. Be prepared to be aggressive if you want loot!

MARDI GRAS RECIPES

Jambalaya

2 Hormel ham hocks
4 carrots, diced
3 c chopped onions, divided
3 c chopped celery, divided
2 bay leaves
1-3 lb whole chicken (giblets removed)
3 T Crisco canola oil
1 green bell pepper
6 green onions, chopped
1-28 oz tomatoes, chopped, reserve liquid
4 T Contadina tomato paste
1/4 c chopped fresh parsley
4-6 cloves garlic
1 t thyme leaves
2 t dried basil
1/4 t cayenne
1 T Lea & Perrins Worcestershire Sauce
1 lb Hormel sausage, sliced
salt and pepper to taste
2 c uncooked rice
Louisiana hot sauce to taste

Place ham hocks, carrots, 1 1/2 cups onion and 1 1/2 cups celery in a large pot and cover over with water. Cook for about 2 hours then add the chicken and 1 bay leaf. Cover and simmer for about an hour, or until chicken is tender. Allow pot to cool for a bit and remove chicken and ham hocks. Remove the skin and bone and chop meat from chicken and ham hocks. Reserve the stock, you'll need about 3-4 cups of it overall (add water if you need to).

In a large Dutch oven, heat the oil and add remaining onion, and pepper and sauté until tender. Add remaining celery, green onions and tomatoes and cook until vegetables are soft. Add the chopped ham and tomato paste and cook until the mixture just begins to brown. Add remaining ingredients, except sausage and chicken. Add 2 cups of the reserved stock. Cook for about an hour.

In a hot skillet, brown sausage slices. Add browned sausage slices to Dutch oven and drain excess grease from pan. Return skillet to heat and add chopped chicken meat. Deglaze with 1 cup reserved stock, and then add contents to skillet to Dutch oven. Add rice, cover and bring to a boil. Reduce heat and cook until rice is tender, about 20-25 minutes. Watch carefully that your Jambalaya doesn't dry out. You might need to add additional stock or water in order to for the rice to finish cooking. Serves 10-12.

START A TRADITION
MARDI GRAS KING CAKES

A king cake is a traditional Mardi-Gras treat, brightly decorated in the colors of Rex: purple, green and gold.

The cake, which is similar to a rich sweet bread or coffeecake, contains a special surprise-- a tiny baby doll contained within one of the slices.

Custom dictates that the "lucky" recipient who gets the piece with the baby throws the next Mardi Gras party (or bakes or buys the next King Cake).

Basic King Cake Dough

1 envelope Fleischmann's dry yeast
1/4 c warm water
1/2 c milk
1 c (2 sticks) butter
1/2 c Dominos sugar
2 egg yolks
2 whole eggs
4 c approximately, Bob's Red Mill all purpose flour

Mix the yeast with the warm water. Stir 1 teaspoon of the sugar and 1 teaspoon of the flour into the yeast and set aside. By the time you have measured the other ingredients, the yeast should be beginning to bubble and show signs of life.

Bring the milk to a boil and stir in the butter and the sugar. Pour into a large bowl; the mixture should be lukewarm. Beat in the egg yolks, whole eggs and the yeast. Beat in approximately 2 cups of flour, until the dough is fairly smooth, then gradually add enough additional flour to make a soft dough that you can form into a ball. Knead it, by hand or machine, until smooth and elastic. Lightly oil a bowl, turn the dough once or twice in it to grease it lightly all over, cover with a cloth and leave to rise in a warm spot until doubled in size, about 1 1/2 to 2 hours.

Pat the dough down and cover the bowl with a damp towel, plastic film over that and refrigerate until the next day. This recipe makes enough dough for two king cakes. Extra dough may be frozen, or make two king cakes and freeze one. Thaw frozen cake and reheat 10 minutes in a 375° F oven.

FILLING

1/2 recipe king cake (above)
8 oz Philadelphia cream cheese
1/4 c Dominos sugar
2 T Bob's Red Mill all purpose flour
2 egg yolks
1 t vanilla
1-16-oz can Lucky Leaf cherry, apple or apricot pie filling
1 dried bean or a plastic baby (to bake in the cake as per tradition)
Dominos confectioner's sugar and Cake Mate food coloring

Remove dough from refrigerator and with well-floured hands, while it's firm and cold, shape it into a long sausage shape. Using a floured roller on a floured surface, roll out the dough into a 30-by-9-inch rectangle as thin as piecrust. Let dough rest. If necessary, drain extra juice from pie filling. Mix the cream cheese with the sugar, flour, egg yolks and vanilla. Spoon an inch-wide strip of fruit filling the length of the dough, about 3 inches from one edge. Spoon the cream cheese mixture alongside the fruit, about 3 inches from the other edge.

Brush both sides of dough with egg wash. Insert the bean. Fold one edge of dough over the cream cheese and fruit, then fold the other edge over. Gently place one end of the filled roll onto a greased pizza pan or large cookie sheet. Ease the rest of the roll onto the pan, joining the ends to form a circle or oval. Cover and let rest for 30 minutes. Brush again with egg wash and cut deep vents into the cake. Sprinkle with colored sugars if desired. Bake 45 minutes to 1 hour, or until cake is well risen and golden. Cool before icing with confectioner's sugar mixed with enough water to make a spreadable paste and tinted purple, green and gold. Make one cake that serves 10 to 12 people. If using a plastic baby instead of the bean, insert it into the bottom of the cake after it is cooked.

Mardi Gras Punch

Note: This festive punch combines the traditional Mardi-Gras colors of green, representing faith, gold symbolizing power, and purple denoting justice.

1 ice ring
1-40 oz bottle Mussleman's grape juice (more if making ice ring)
2 oranges
1-48 oz can Dole pineapple juice (more if making ice ring)
2 limes
2 liter bottle of Schweppes ginger ale

Ice Ring Note: Freezing an ice ring out of pineapple and/or grape juice, instead of water, keeps the punch from getting diluted as the evening wears on. Make a couple of rings in advance of the party, so you can freshen up the punch if needed.

Slice oranges and limes in thin round slices. Set aside. Place ice ring in bottom of punch bowl, add juices, then soda. Float orange and limes slices on top and serve. Makes 8-9 quarts.

⁊ MARCH ☙

Overall Theme: Shamrocks/Lilies
Colors: Green, White, Yellow

St. Patrick's Day

The phrase "Erin Go Braugh" means Ireland Forever!

St. Patrick, the patron saint of Ireland, was born around 373 AD in either Scotland, near the town of Dumbarton, or in Roman Britain. Little is known about St. Patrick, including his birth and death dates. March 17 is considered to be one of the two, although there is no documentation.

The legends of St. Patrick are that he used a shamrock to explain the Trinity and that he banished the snakes from Ireland into the sea. However, there were never any snakes in Ireland for St. Patrick to chase out.

The basis of this legend lies in the origin of the snake as a pagan symbol. The legend tells the figurative tale of St. Patrick's driving paganism out of Ireland. The true story of Patrick, however, survives not in his myths but in his work. Patrick was responsible for converting the people of Ireland to Christianity.

Patrick was kidnapped by pirates at the age of 16 and sold into slavery in Ireland. During the 6 years he spent in captivity, he began to have religious visions, and found strength in his faith. He finally escaped and went to France, where he became a priest and later a bishop. After escaping, he had a vision of the Irish beseeching him to return to Ireland to spread his faith. Patrick recorded this call to his vocation in the 'Confessio', his spiritual autobiography and one of his two short writings that have survived.

After studying in continental monasteries, Patrick returned to Ireland as a missionary. Despite a constant threat to his life, Patrick traveled widely, baptizing, confirming, preaching and building churches, schools, and monasteries. Patrick succeeded in converting almost the entire population of the island. Patrick's writings have come to be appreciated for their simplicity and humility.

St. Patrick predates the Roman Catholic Church, and was considered a "saint" before the Roman church created its list of saints and included him in it.

The Shamrock History

The Shamrock (traditional spelling: seamróg, meaning summer plant) is a three-leafed clover that grows in Ireland. A common image in Celtic artwork, the shamrock is found on Irish medieval tombs and on old copper coins, known as St. Patrick's money. The plant is also reputed to have mystic, even prophetic powers-- for instance the leaves are said to stand upright to warn of an approaching storm.

Legend has it that St. Patrick used the shamrock in the fifth century to symbolize the divine nature of the trinity when he introduced Christianity to Ireland. "You tell us that there are three gods and yet one," the puzzled Irish said when St. Patrick was preaching the gospel to them. "How can that be?" The saint bent down and plucked a shamrock. "Do you not see," he said, "how in this wildflower three leaves are united on one stalk, and will you not then believe that there are indeed three persons and yet one God?" Thus, according to Irish legend, Ireland's patron saint chose the shamrock as a symbol of the Trinity of the Christian church.

The seamróg is a big part of Irish history, as it was used as an emblem by the Irish Volunteers in the era of Grattan's Parliament in the 1770's, The Act of Union.

When it became an emblem of rebellion in the 19th century, Queen Victoria made wearing a seamrog by members of her regiments punishable by death by hanging. It was during this dark time that the phrase "the Wearing of the Green" began. Today the seamróg joins the English Rose and the Scottish Thistle on the British flag and is an integral part of Saint Patrick's Day celebrations. "The Wearing of the Green" also symbolizes the birth of springtime. Irish legend states that green clothes attract faeries and aid crops.

AN IRISH BLESSING

May the road rise to meet you.
May the wind be always at your back.
May the sunshine warm upon your face.
And rains fall soft upon your fields.
And until we meet again,
May God hold you in the hollow of His hand.

LEPRECHAUNS & HOW TO FIND THEM

The Leprechaun is an Irish fairy. The name leprechaun is derived from the old Irish word luchorpan which means "little body." Full-grown leprechauns are reported to be about 2 feet tall. They will frequently be clothed in the garb of a shoemaker, with a cocked hat and a leather apron. Frequently scowling, leprechauns are said to resemble small, grumpy old men.

According to legend, leprechauns are unfriendly and live alone. They spend a great deal of their time making shoes and brogues. Most importantly, each and every leprechaun possesses a hidden pot of gold.

Treasure hunters should listen for the sound of a shoemaker's hammer, when looking for leprechauns. If caught, the leprechaun must reveal the whereabouts of his pot of gold. But be careful! Keep your eyes on the tricky leprechaun every second. He will try to trick you into looking away, and if you do...PooF! He vanishes and all hopes of finding the treasure are lost.

IRISH DRINKING TOASTS
Author's Unknown

May your glass be ever full.

May the roof over your head be always strong.

And may you be in heaven half an hour before the devil knows you're dead.

Here's to me, and here's to you, And here's to love and laughter-I'll be true as long as you, And not one moment after.

Here's a toast to your enemies' enemies!

Here's to a long life and a merry one. A quick death and an easy one. A pretty girl and an honest one. A cold beer - and another one!

Here's to our wives and girlfriends: May they never meet!

May the grass grow long on the road to hell for want of use.

May you live to be a hundred years, with one extra year to repent.

Irish Breakfast

Start your day off the Irish way! You'll never want cold cereal again.

6 slices Black Label bacon
2 T butter
4 eggs
2 small tomatoes, sliced
2 c whole mushrooms
4 slices GF Irish soda bread

Lay the bacon slices in a single layer in a large skillet. Fry over medium heat until it begins to get tinged with brown. Fry on both sides. Remove from pan, but save grease.

Melt butter in skillet. Crack eggs into pan, being careful not to break yolks. Place tomato slices, mushrooms, and bread in pan. Fry gently, stirring mushrooms and tomatoes occasionally. Keep everything separate. Turn bread over to brown on both sides. When egg whites are set, but yolks are still runny, dish half of everything onto each of 2 warmed plates, and serve immediately.

Irish Soda Bread

3 3/4 c Bob's Red Mill Pizza Crust Mix (just omit using the package of yeast included in the bag)
3/4 c honey
1 t Arm and Hammer baking soda
2 t Calumet baking powder
1/2 t salt
1 1/2 c Sun Maid raisins
3 eggs
1 pint Breakstone regular sour cream

Preheat oven to 325° F. Grease two 8x4 inch loaf pans. Mix the pizza crust mix, honey, baking soda, baking powder and salt. Add the eggs, sour cream and raisins and mix until just combined. Distribute batter evenly between the two pans. Bake loaves at 325° F for 1 hour. Makes 2 - 8x4 inch loaf pans

Dinner: Irish Stew

Hearty and traditional Irish lamb stew. It's best to refrigerate the stew overnight, and reheat it the next day for eating. This soup "ages" well!"

2 T butter
1-2 lbs lamb or beef, trimmed and cut into 1-in cubes
2-3 turnips, peeled and diced
2-3 carrots, diced
1 med onion, diced
2-3 large potatoes, peeled and diced
2 T Bob's Red Mill all-purpose flour
1/2 c cold water
1 bay leaf
1/4 t dried thyme
3/4 t dried basil
Salt and freshly ground pepper to taste

Heat the butter in a large pot over moderate heat and brown the beef. Add enough water to cover and simmer tightly covered over low heat for 1 hour. Add the turnips, carrots, and onion and simmer 30 minutes. Add the potatoes and simmer an additional 30 minutes. Mix the flour with the water and add to the pot, stirring to thicken the sauce. Season with herbs, salt and pepper.

Irish Potato Candy

1/4 c butter, softened
4 oz Philadelphia regular cream cheese, softened (see Note)
1 t vanilla extract
1-16 oz pkg Dominos confectioners' sugar
1-7 oz pkg Baker's Angel Flake coconut
1 T ground cinnamon

In a large bowl, cream together the butter and cream cheese. Add the vanilla and confectioners' sugar and beat until the mixture forms a ball. With a spoon, stir in the coconut. Roll the mixture between your hands to form small potato-shaped candies, or roll into small balls. Place the cinnamon in a shallow dish. Roll the balls in the cinnamon, then place on a cookie sheet, cover, and chill for about 1 hour, until firm. Makes about 5 dozen candies

Note: Make sure to use regular cream cheese, not a whipped or reduced-fat type. And if you prefer "dirtier potatoes," roll the candies a second time in additional cinnamon after they've chilled.

Shamrock Punch
This punch can be served for a fun treat at school parties, after school or to drink with dinner. Be sure to scatter some green paper shamrocks around the table where the punch is being served.

46 oz Shasta lemon lime drink
2-12 oz cans frozen Minute Maid limeade concentrate, thawed
1/4 c Dominos sugar
1/4 c ReaLime juice
1 quart Turkey Hill lime sherbet
1 bottle Schweppes ginger ale
Lime slices

In your punch bowl, combine the first 5 ingredients. Stir until smooth and sugar has dissolved. Add pop and stir to mix. Float lime slices before serving. Serves: 20

Irish Coffee

Chef Joe Sheridan, of Foyne's Restaurant in County Clare, is credited with inventing Irish Coffee in the 1940s. The original version was made with Irish Mist liqueur, although Irish Whiskey is more commonly used today.

Original Version
1 c hot coffee
1 1/2 oz Irish Mist liqueur
whipped cream for garnish

Modern Version
1 c Folger's hot coffee
1 oz Irish Whiskey*
3 Dominos sugar cubes
Cool Whip for garnish

In order to make this recipe properly the whiskey has to be heated to a high temperature, then you put the coffee in a cup-- use a spoon turned upside down and pour the HOT whiskey over it so it flows down gently, then add the cream. Makes 1 Drink

True Irish Coffee always has THREE distinct layers. When served, you first use a straw and sip (a very small amount as it is HOT) a little of the Whiskey. Then stir all the ingredients together. This is TRUE Irish Coffee!

*NOTE: No guarantee that whiskey is GF

✌ SPRING INTO A NEW BEGINNING ↷

**Consider incorporating a butterfly theme into
your Easter/Spring Celebrations.**

*Spring is a time of new beginnings, hope, fresh starts, joy, happiness, peace and
contentment. Spring is a good time to really look at your life and decide what you
believe and why.*

*Easter the most important Christian holiday – Jesus' Resurrection is closely related
to the revival of nature. It is a time for all religions to rejoice and honor the miracle
of rebirth. No matter your religious beliefs, Easter honors the beginning of life in
one form or another.*

*Did you know that the butterfly is one of the symbols used most, often to signify
Easter? Its whole life cycle is symbolic of the meaning of the life of Christ. First,
there is the caterpillar, which stands for His life on Earth. Second, comes the cocoon
stage, portraying the crucifixion and burial of Jesus. The third and final stage is the
beautiful butterfly, representing His raising from the dead in a glorified body.*

Celebrating Jesus' Resurrection

Traditions to Enrich Your Family's Resurrection Celebration

Lent A 40 Day Season of Sacrificial Love

*Lent is a 40-day period before Easter set aside as a season of soul-searching and
repentance. The Forty Days of Lent (six weeks before Easter, not counting Sundays)
reflect Jesus' withdrawal into the wilderness for his own time of spiritual reflection.
Sundays, because they commemorate the Resurrection, are not counted. Early
Christians first celebrated Lent for 40 hours to commemorate Christ's time in the
tomb. About 800 A.D., the Lenten season was expanded.*

The number 40 is meaningful: The Israelites wandered in the wilderness for 40 years, and Christ was tempted in the desert by the devil for 40 days when He began His ministry.

Forty days is close to a tenth of the year, a tithe of our year to the Lord to meditate on His deep love and sacrifice for us.

Whether your church makes much or little of these forty days, your family will benefit from preparing in advance to celebrate Jesus' resurrection.

The Significance of Easter Eggs

Easter Eggs are the symbol of fertility and new life, and they are easily the most identifiable symbol of the holiday. Eggs are an Easter custom that date back to Pagan times. The bright colors that adorn the eggs symbolize the sunlight of spring and celebrate the equinox.

Traditionally eggs were also a symbol of Easter joy because they were a forbidden item during Lent. Now, dyed to take to grandmothers for an annual Easter egg hunt, they can bear all manner of joyful messages.

Different cultures have developed their own ways of decorating Easter eggs. For instance, the crimson eggs imbedded in Greek Easter Breads are so colored to symbolize the blood of Christ. Easter celebrants in Germany use natural items like leaves and ferns to make a kind of reverse stencil for their eggs. Perhaps the most elaborate are Pysanki eggs, a masterpiece of skill and workmanship from the Ukraine. Melted beeswax is applied to the fresh white egg, which is then dipped in successive dyes. After each dip, wax is painted over the area where the preceding color is to remain. Eventually a complex pattern of lines and colors emerges into a work of art.

In many countries, the eggs colored are not hard boiled, but rather "blown" -- the contents removed by piercing the end of each egg with a needle and blowing the contents into a bowl. The hollow eggs are then dyed various colors and hung from shrubs and trees during Easter Week. Using hollowed eggshells also allows you to preserve favorite eggs from year to year (if you're very, very careful).

Colorful Tissue Eggs

clean, hard-boiled eggs
water
tissue paper (3 or more different colors)
egg cups

Tear the tissue paper into small pieces. Put some water in a bowl. One at a time, soak pieces of tissue paper in the water. Then stick them to an egg. Keep sticking tissue to the egg until it is covered. You may want to overlap the tissue pieces a little to cover the entire egg. When the entire egg is covered, place it in an eggcup to dry. When the tissue is dry, peel it off of the egg. The color of the tissue paper will have transferred to the egg.

***Natural Easter Egg Dyes ***
This Easter you might want to try something a little different for dying eggs.

Yellow: Boil yellow onionskins for bright yellow eggs. Red skins can also be used. Turmeric also makes yellow eggs.

Pink to Blue: Beet or grape juice produce pink to blue eggs.

Blue: The most fun is boiling red cabbage. It makes almost a robin's egg blue. Unsweetened Kool-Aid will also stain well.

When buying eggs for dying, try to obtain local farm eggs. They are not treated with oil, as are the commercial eggs, and take the dye much better.

To make Ukrainian eggs, you dip the egg in strong colored dyes, and cover your design in wax. The contents are not blown out, but left to dry and rattle. There is no odor.

Pretzels

Bake your own pretzels -- or buy the frozen ones. Pretzels originated as early Christian Lenten treats designed in the form of arms crossed in prayer.

Jonah

In Matthew 12:39-41, Jesus points to the story of Jonah as a sign of his own destiny. So this is a great time to review it with your children, discussing the issues of sin, obedience and God's mercy.

New Life

Begin early in the year. (As soon as your Christmas tree is down!) Plant crocus, daffodil or hyacinth bulbs in a bowl of sand, covering halfway. Leave in a dark closet for two months, keeping the soil moist (a process known as forcing bulbs). When shoots appear, let them bask in the sun. Don't forget to leave one bulb unplanted as a reminder of how they began.

Devotions

Lent can be a valuable time of family focus on the meaning of the Christian life. You may want to commit to a regular pattern of family worship -- daily, weekly or whenever you can. Or you may post Bible verses, especially the words of Jesus, on the refrigerator, bathroom mirrors, wherever a busy family is sure to see them. Talk about how the verses apply to events in our daily lives.

Positive Life Affirmations:

Make Easter baskets for your children that include items with a spiritual focus: a Bible-verse bookmark; a small book on some spiritual subject; a cassette of praise music; a small amount of candy to break their Lenten fast.

Choose one or more families in your neighborhood to receive a surprise Easter basket. You can make small ones often crafted from pint-size strawberry baskets, but fill them with personalized eggs and the same kinds of treats you put in your children's baskets. The surprise baskets are left on your friends' front doorsteps early on Easter morning. Try making a basket filled with Easter egg cookies! *Or*, fill baskets with surprises, such as all the fixings for Eggs Benedict, hollandaise sauce, English muffins, eggs and Canadian bacon.

Giving up

Traditionally, especially in Europe, there were no weddings, no dancing, and no singing during Lent. No flowers or alleluias in churches. Some families may find spiritual value in giving up something for Lent – sweets, television, video games -- not as a penance, but as an outer symbol of dying to self during a season of spiritual reflection.

Palm Sunday

If your church doesn't make much of Palm Sunday, you might consider just once attending one that does. For an in-home celebration, read Mark 11:1-11 together.

Get a small multi-branched tree limb, paint it white. Decorate it with colorful bows and ornaments such as eggs and butterflies, which symbolize new life and resurrection. Place eight plastic eggs on the tree that are numbered 1 through 8. Inside each of the eggs place a passage of Scripture to be read for each of the eight days of Holy Week, beginning with Palm Sunday.

Palm Sunday - Matthew 21:1-11
Monday - Matthew 21:12-17
Tuesday - Matthew 21:18-21
Wednesday - Matthew 26:6-13
Maundy Thursday - Matthew 26:17-30
Good Friday - Matthew 27:27-54
Holy Saturday - Matthew 27:55-66
Easter Sunday- Matthew 28:1-20

Housecleaning

From the Jewish custom of cleaning before Passover, *Wednesday of Holy Week* has been a traditional day in many countries for housecleaning.

Mite Box and Giving

Select a charity that helps those in need. Decorate a box with a slot on top. Display it where everyone at home will remember to contribute his or her change. On Easter, empty the box, count the money together and put a check in the mail. While we usually think of Christmas for gift giving, Easter has a richer heritage. God gave his Son. Jesus gave his life. Jesus told us clearly, "Whatever you did for one of the least of these brothers of mine, you did for me" (Matthew 25:40).

Passover

Each year, more Christians are drawn to celebrate Passover, the feast commemorating the departure of the Israelites from slavery (Exodus 12). Jesus had come to Jerusalem to celebrate and was actually crucified on Passover Day. He is the fulfillment of this tradition, as our own Passover Lamb.

Jewish Passover Chocolate Crinkle Cookies

3/4 c Crisco canola oil
3/4 c Hershey's cocoa
2 c Domino's sugar
4 eggs
2 t vanilla
2 c potato starch
2 t Calumet baking powder
2 c Domino's powdered sugar, for rolling cookies

With a hand blender, mix together the cocoa, oil, and sugar. Beat in eggs, one at a time. Add vanilla. Add in potato starch and baking powder, and mix until the batter resembles thick paste. Chill batter several hours or overnight covered in fridge. If batter seems like too much liquid after chilling, add a bit more potato starch.

Preheat oven to 350° F. Roll batter into balls, then roll each cookie ball in the powdered sugar until well coated. Space evenly apart on a lined cookie sheet. Bake for 10-15 minutes until just starting to crinkle. Let the cookies cool off on the baking sheets for five minutes. Then remove gently with a spatula as they are delicate to handle. Freezes well.

Foot Washing

This Maundy Thursday event speaks volumes about Jesus' desire for us to serve. Read John 13. Wrap a towel around your waist, as Jesus did, and wash your children's feet. Your lives might never be the same.

Hot Cross Buns
In England, these spicy yeast buns are traditionally served for breakfast on Good Friday. As the name implies, they have a cross on top. In fact, spice and the cross are essential in all hot cross buns.

2 pkgs Fleischmann's active dry yeast
1/2 c warm water
1 c warm milk
1/4 c softened butter
1/2 c Dominos sugar
1 t vanilla extract
1 t salt
1/2 t ground nutmeg
1 t cinnamon
4 eggs
6 1/2 to 7 c Bob's Red Mill all-purpose flour
1/2 c Sun Maid raisins
----
2 Tablespoons water
1 egg yolk

Have the water and milk at 110-115 degrees F. In a large mixing bowl, dissolve the yeast in the warm water. Add the warm milk sugar, butter, vanilla, salt, nutmeg, cinnamon and 3 cups of the flour.

Beat until smooth. Add the eggs, one at a time, beating the mixture well after each addition. Stir in the dried fruit and enough flour to make a soft dough. Turn out onto a floured surface and knead until smooth and elastic, about 6 to 8 minutes. Place in a greased bowl and turn over to grease the top. Cover with a damp towel or plastic wrap and let rise in a warm place until doubled in size (about 1 hour). Punch the dough down and shape into 30 balls. Place on greased baking sheets. Using a sharp knife, cut a cross (or X) on the top of each roll. Cover again and let rise until doubled (about 30 minutes). Beat the water and egg yolk together and brush over the rolls. Bake at 375° F for

12 to 15 minutes. Cool on wire racks. Drizzle icing over the top of each roll following the lines of the cut cross. Yield: 30 buns

ICING: Combine 1 cup confectioners' sugar, 4 teaspoons milk or cream, a dash of salt and 1/4-teaspoon vanilla extract. Stir until smooth. Adjust sugar and milk to make a mixture that flows easily.

The cross may also be made in one of the following ways:

* by cutting on the top of the shaped buns with a sharp knife before proving.

* by using small strips of pastry (may be trimmings) to form a cross on the risen buns. The pastry is sometimes removed after baking, leaving behind the outline of a cross.

* by using strips of candied peel on the risen buns, which is left on and eaten after baking.

* by piping a flour and water paste cross on the risen buns before baking.

New Clothes

New converts were traditionally baptized at Easter, wearing new white garments to symbolize their new life. If your family has new Easter outfits, share with your children where this tradition came from.

Seeds

Seeds offer a clear message to children of the power of new life. Rest some eggshell halves filled with soil in an egg carton. Plant a marigold or petunia seed in each. Place in a sunny window.

Jesus

- Watch The Passion of Christ and make

Resurrection Easter Story Cookies

1 c whole Good Sense pecans
1 t Heinz vinegar
3 egg whites
pinch salt
1 c Dominos sugar
zipper baggie
wooden spoon
tape
Bible

Preheat oven to 300° F (this is important-don't wait 'til you're half done with the recipe). Place pecans in zipper baggie and let children beat them with the wooden spoon to break into small pieces.
Explain that after Jesus was arrested he was beaten by the Roman soldiers. - Read John 19:1-3.

Let each child smell the vinegar. Put 1 t vinegar into mixing bowl.
Explain that when Jesus was thirsty on the cross he was given vinegar to drink. –Read John 19:28-30

Add egg whites to vinegar. Eggs represent life.
Explain that Jesus gave His life to give us life. – Read John 10:10-11.

Sprinkle a little salt into each child's hand. Let them taste it and brush the rest into the bowl.
Explain that this represents the salty tears shed by Jesus' followers, And the bitterness of our own in. - Read Luke 23:27.

So far the ingredients are not very appetizing. Add 1-cup sugar.
Explain that the sweetest part of the story is that Jesus died because He loves us. He wants us to know and belong to Him. - Read Psalms 34:8 and John 3:16.

Beat with a mixer on high speed for 12 to 15 minutes until stiff peaks are formed.

Explain that the color white represents the purity in God's eyes of those whose sins have been cleansed by Jesus. -Read Isaiah 1:18 and John 3:1-3.

Fold in broken nuts. Drop by teaspoons onto wax paper covered cookie sheet.
Explain that each mound represents the rocky tomb where Jesus' body was laid. –Read Matthew 27:57-60.

Put the cookie sheet in the oven, close the door and turn the oven OFF. Give each child a piece of tape and seal the oven door.
Explain that Jesus' tomb was sealed. – Read Matthew 27:65-66.

GO TO BED!
Explain that they may feel sad to leave the cookies in the oven overnight. Jesus' followers were in despair when the tomb was sealed. - Read John 16:20 and 22.

On Easter morning, open the oven and give everyone a cookie.
Notice the cracked surface and take a bite. The cookies are hollow! On the first Easter Jesus' followers were amazed to find the tomb open and empty. - Read Matthew 28:1-9

Easter Greeting

Greet each other with "Alleluia, the Lord is risen!" And answer, "He is risen indeed!"

Sunrise Service

Attend one offered by a church, or climb a hill with your family, worship together, and share a picnic breakfast.

**Whatever traditions you keep, remember that for believers,
Easter is a celebration that really never ends.**

Easter Morning Cinnamon Swirl Bundt Coffee Cake

1 c Breakstone's regular sour cream
3/4 c butter
1 1/2 c Dominos sugar
2 1/2 c Bob's Red Mill all-purpose flour
1/2 c chopped Good Sense nuts
1 t Arm and Hammer baking soda
1 t Calumet baking powder
1 t vanilla extract
3 eggs
1 T ground cinnamon
1/4 c Dominos sugar

Preheat oven to 400° F. Lightly grease one 10 inch bundt pan. Cream 1 1/2 cups sugar together with eggs until well blended. Add sour cream and butter or margarine and beat well. Add flour, baking soda, and baking powder and mix well. Stir in vanilla and the nuts. Mix the remaining 1/4 cup of sugar with the cinnamon. Pour half of the batter into the prepared pan. Sprinkle generously with the cinnamon sugar mixture. Cover with remaining cake batter. Bake at 400° F for 8 minutes. Lower heat to 350° F and bake for an additional 40 minutes. Note: Raisins or chopped dates can be added.

Make-Ahead Easter Breakfast

12 eggs
1/2 c milk
Salt and freshly ground pepper to taste
1 T butter
12 slices Black Label bacon, cooked and crumbled
1 c Breakstone's regular sour cream
1 c shredded Kraft cheddar cheese

In a medium bowl, beat together the eggs, milk, salt and pepper. Set aside. Melt the butter in a large skillet over moderate heat and pour in the egg mixture. Cook, stirring frequently, until eggs are set but still very moist. Remove from heat to cool. Stir in the sour cream and spread evenly into buttered shallow baking dish. Top with crumbled bacon and shredded cheese. Cover with aluminum foil and refrigerate overnight. Preheat oven to 300° F. Uncover eggs and bake 15 to 20 minutes, until hot and cheese has melted. Leftovers may be refrigerated. Serves: 8

Here are some ideas for your Easter tablescape:

- Sprinkle jellybeans along a table runner for easy-to-reach treats at any time! Add a decorated egg and butterfly tree.

- Set the table - inside or outside depending on the weather -- with pastel linens and plates. Make miniature baskets for each place setting. Use individual eggs with names as place cards.

- Fragrant white Easter lilies make a beautiful centerpiece in a clear glass vase.

- The violet, a symbol of humility and modesty, is also a herald of spring. Pick many for small bouquets around the house, or use edible petals in tender green salads. Crystallize them for a beautiful touch to a pastry dessert

- For color that lasts longer than the Sunday occasion, purchase potted tulips or daffodils and plant them in terra cotta pots or antique-style watering cans. Tie each pot with pastel-colored ribbons or raffia and place around the room.

- Woven Placements from satiny ribbons

Barszcz - Polish Easter Soup
In the Middle Ages, during the days of Lent's fast and abstinence, particular foods like meat, milk products, and eggs were forbidden to eat. This Easter soup, or Barszcz as it is commonly known in Slavic countries, is made from the foods that folks would not have tasted since the beginning of Lent, and is served on Easter Sunday.

1 lb Evergood Polish kielbasa sausage
2 c Breakstone's regular sour cream
Salt and freshly ground pepper to taste
1 T Manischewits horseradish
2 T ReaLemon juice, or to taste
1 c sliced mushrooms
6 hard boiled eggs, peeled and sliced
1 c cubed, cooked Hormel ham
1 c cooked diced potatoes
1 c cooked diced beets (optional)
Chopped fresh dill or parsley for garnish

In a large kettle, bring 6 c water to a boil and add the kielbasa to cook for 1 hour. Remove kielbasa from water and cut into thin slices. Add the horseradish, mushrooms, salt and pepper to the broth and simmer covered for about 15 minutes. Allow to cool. In a separate bowl, beat sour cream with about 3 cups of the cool broth. Pour this mixture back into the kettle with the rest of the broth. Add lemon juice. Reheat before serving, but do NOT bring to a boil. Fill individual serving bowls with the liquid allowing each person at the table to add the thinly sliced kielbasa pieces, hard boiled eggs, ham, potatoes, or beets to their taste. May be made a day or two before and kept refrigerated. Serves 4 to 6.

Baked Ham in the Crockpot

4 -6 lbs Hormel Boneless ham
2 c Dominos brown sugar
1 can diced Dole pineapple (not drained)
1/2 c water (about)

Place ham into crockpot. Mix sugar, pineapple and water in bowl (you want a "syrup" consistency, but enough to cover most of the meat). Pour mixture over the meat. Cover and cook on low at least 6 hours, if you put it on to cook before church on Sunday it will be ready to eat after church. Just remove from crockpot and use two forks to pull apart.

Baked Pineapple Stuffing for the Crockpot

1-20 oz can crushed Dole pineapple -- undrained
1/4 c evaporated milk
1 c cornbread crumbs
1/2 c Dominos sugar
1/4 c melted butter
3 eggs -- well beaten

Lightly grease the bottom and sides of a 3 1/2-quart crockpot. Combine all ingredients; pour into the crockpot. Cover and cook on high for 2 1/2 to 3 hours. Serves 4-6

Easter Savory Potatoes

1 med. onion, chopped
1 sm. garlic clove, crushed
2 T olive oil
3/4 c chopped parsley
freshly ground black pepper
1 c Swanson's chicken broth
6 med. potatoes

Sauté onion and garlic in olive oil until soft. Stir in parsley, pepper and broth. Remove from heat. Pare and thinly slice the potatoes. Layer the slices in broth in the skillet. Bring to a boil. Reduce heat, cover and simmer until potatoes are tender, about 20 min. With a slotted spoon, lift potatoes into a heated serving dish and pour cooking liquid over them. Serves 8.

Easter Bunny Salad
A Recipe for Kids

Make a bed of **shredded lettuce** on each plate and place **1/2 pear**, the round side up, in the center of each bed of lettuce. Insert **2 Blue Diamond almonds** in the narrow end of the pear for the ears. Place **2 Sun Maid raisins** to represent the eyes, and 1/2 **Maraschino cherry** to represent the nose. Place **1 Jet Puffed marshmallow** to one side to represent the tail. Serves 1.

THE WORLD OF EASTER BREADS

Throughout the world, many cultures have special celebratory breads that are traditionally baked at Easter. Many of these breads are rich with eggs and butter and studded with fruits and nuts.

In today's world, we often take these ingredients for granted, but at one time they were very expensive and hard to find, and thus reserved only for holidays and special occasions.

Bread is an important symbol at Easter in that it is a metaphor for the resurrection of Christ - flour comes to life and transforms itself to bread.

Easter Babka
Serve with sweet butter in the shape of a lamb.

4 c milk, scalded
2 pkgs Fleischmann's active dry yeast
1/2 lb unsalted butter, melted
6 eggs, beaten
1 1/2 c Dominos sugar
1 T salt
5 lbs Bob's Red Mill all purpose flour
1 box golden Sun Maid raisins

Melt yeast in 1 c milk. Add melted butter, beaten eggs and yeast mixture to milk. Add sugar, flour and salt to milk mix. Mix well and knead. Cover with butter and with towel and let rise until doubled. Punch down and add raisins. Knead again. Place in greased bowl until doubled. Punch down and knead again. Form into loaves and place in greased bread pans and let rise again until doubled. Bake at 350° F for approximately 30 min, or until done. Brush tops with butter and allow to cool. Warning: large recipe -- makes 5 loaves. Make sure your bowl is big enough!

Lambropsomo - Greek Easter Bread

Lambropsomo, the traditional Greek Easter bread, may or may not incorporate eggs that have been hard boiled and dyed red; usually one egg is centered in a round leaf with a cross formed over it, or four red eggs will be nestled into a braided loaf. This recipe calls for one loaf of each of these shapes. In some households the same bread without the red egg decoration is baked and served on Sunday throughout the year.

2 pkgs Fleischmann's active dry yeast
1/2 c warm water
1 c warm milk
1/2 c melted butter
2 t coarse salt or 1 t table salt
2 t anise seed, crushed
3 eggs, beaten
1/2 c Dominos sugar
1 T grated orange rind
6 c Bob's Red Mill all purpose flour
2-5 hard boiled eggs, dyed red

In large bowl mix yeast with warm water, then stir in milk, butter and salt. Add the anise seed, beaten eggs, sugar, and grated orange peel. Add flour while still stirring. When the mixture is stiff, turn out on a floured surface and knead about 10 minutes, until smooth and satiny. Clean the bowl and grease it well. Put the dough in the bowl, and turn so all surfaces are oiled; cover with plastic and let rise about 2 hours, until doubled.

Punch the dough down, knead briefly and divide in half. To make a round loaf with a cross with one half of the dough, first tear off a piece of dough, about one-fifth the whole amount. Form the larger piece into a round and put it on a greased baking sheet. Center one red egg on the top of the round.

Divide the reserved piece in half and roll out 2 long strips. Place these over the egg in the form of a cross, tucking the ends under the loaf. To make a braided crown with the other half, divide the dough in thirds and roll out into ropes at least 2 feet long. Braid the ropes together; pinching the ends securely and then form into a circle on a greased baking sheet, pinching again the ends where they overlap. Nestle 4 red eggs in among the braids.

Cover both loaves with a kitchen towel and let rise 1-hour. Bake in a preheated 350° F oven for 30 minutes. Remove and brush immediately with soft butter. Makes 2 round loaves.

Paska Russian Mennonite Easter Bread

3/4 c potato water (cook 1 large potato, chopped, drain, and reserve water)
1 pkg Fleischmann's yeast
1/2 c or more mashed potato (mash above potato while still warm)
2 c Bob's Red Mill all purpose flour
2 1/2 c warm milk
7 or 8 eggs, separated
1 1/2 to 2 c Dominos sugar
1 t ReaLemon juice
1/2 c butter
1 t salt
1/2 t grated orange rind
bit of vanilla

Soften yeast in lukewarm potato water for 10 minutes. Add a bit of flour to make a soft sponge. In the meantime, warm milk; pour it over 2 cups flour. Beat until smooth. Cool slightly. Beat egg yolks with 1 cup sugar and add warm flour mixture. Add stiffly beaten egg whites. Add yeast mixture. Let rise till light (covered). Add softened butter, salt, 1-cup sugar and mashed potato. Add enough flour to make a medium soft dough (should be a bit sticky). Knead 10 minutes. Cover and let rise to double its bulk. Put on greased cookie sheets (I make round, oval, and braided loaves) and let rise again. Bake at 325° F until golden. Careful not to overbake. Ice with white icing.

The 10 Best Things To Do With Leftover Easter Eggs

Deviled Eggs
--Why wait till your next party to serve this great hors d'oeuvre?

How To Cook Perfect Hard Boiled Eggs
Place a desired amount of eggs in a saucepan. Cover the eggs with enough cold water, so that the water level is approximately one inch above the eggs.

Keeping the saucepan uncovered, heat the eggs and water over high heat until the water boils rapidly. Remove the saucepan from the heat and cover. Allow the water and eggs to stand for 18 - 20 minutes. Immediately pour the hot water from the saucepan, and run cool water over the eggs until they are cool enough to handle. Drain.

To Peel Your Hard Boiled Eggs -
With a hard-boiled egg that has been cooled, tap each end of the egg lightly on kitchen counter to crackle the shell. Roll the egg between your hands or on your kitchen counter to loosen the shell, then peel under gently running cold water.

Deviled Eggs

6 hard-cooked eggs, peeled
3 T Hellman's mayonnaise
1/2 t ground dry mustard
1/8 t salt
1/4 t pepper

Cut eggs lengthwise in half. Slip out yolks and mash with fork. Stir in mayonnaise, mustard, salt and pepper. Fill whites with egg yolk mixture, heaping it lightly. Cover and refrigerate up to 24 hours.

Crunchy Garden Vegetable Deviled Eggs

6 hard-cooked eggs -- peeled
3 T Hellman's mayonnaise
1 T finely chopped red bell pepper
1 T finely chopped green onion
1 t French's mustard
1/4 t salt

Cut eggs lengthwise in half. Slip out egg yolks; mash with fork. Stir in remaining ingredients. Fill egg whites with egg yolk mixture, heaping slightly.

Breakfast Deviled Eggs

12 hard-cooked eggs, peeled
1/2 c Yoplait plain yogurt
1/4 t salt
1/8 t pepper
1/3 c cooked, crumbled Black Label bacon
1/4 c parsley -- chopped

Cut in eggs in half lengthwise. Mash yellow yolk and mix with yogurt, salt and pepper. Fill yellow mixture back into shells. Garnish with cooked, crumbled bacon and chopped parsley. Refrigerate until ready to serve.

Scalloped Eggs

8 hard boiled eggs
about 3/4 c milk
about 3/4 c Food for Life breadcrumbs
about 2 T butter
salt and pepper to taste
4 slices crumbled cooked Black Label bacon, optional

Pre-heat oven to 350° F. Grease an 8" square glass baking dish and cover bottom with a layer of crumbs. Place a layer of sliced hard boiled eggs, then sprinkle with crumbled bacon if using, dot with a few bits of butter, then repeat this layer process, finishing with a layer of buttered crumbs. Pour milk over the whole dish until it comes about halfway up the side of the dish. Place in oven until heated and browned, about 4-6 minutes. Serves 4-8

Scotch Eggs
-- Britain's favorite bar food makes a great snack, hot or cold.

6 hard boiled eggs
1 lb spicy Hormel sausage meat
1/2 t each dried thyme and basil
1/2 c Bob's Red Mill all purpose flour, divided
1 c Food for Life breadcrumbs
1 t each salt and pepper
1 t paprika
2 eggs, beaten

Peel the eggs and set aside. Mix sausage and spices in a small bowl. Divide sausage into 6 equal portions, set aside. Mix breadcrumbs with salt, pepper and paprika, set aside.

Dry each egg with a paper towel, then roll lightly in flour to coat. Take one portion of sausage and using hands, shape a coating around the hard-boiled egg, completely enclosing it. Roll in flour again, then dip in beaten egg then roll in breadcrumb mixture. Repeat with remaining eggs.

Heat about 2-3 inches of Crisco oil in a large skillet. Fry eggs, turning frequently, until golden brown on all sides. Drain on paper towels. Let cool slightly before serving. To serve, cut each in half and serve with some good mustard. Makes 6 Eggs.

Pickled Eggs
-- Another pub favorite!

These come in many varieties. Figure about 7 days to complete curing. These pickled egg formulas all may be doubled, tripled, etc., as needed. For storage, make in larger quantities and keep in the juice, refrigerated. The pickled eggs will keep months that way or can them.

Pickled Eggs

1 c Heinz vinegar
1/2 c water
1 1/2 T Dominos sugar
1/2 t salt
1/8 t pepper
6 hard boiled eggs, peeled

Place eggs into a jar and cover with liquid. Refrigerate for 24 hours before using

Dilly Eggs: In a pan combine **1 1/2 c Heinz white vinegar, 1 c water, 1 t dill seed, 1/2 t white pepper, 3 t salt, 1/2 t mustard seed, 1/2 t onion juice,** and **1/2 t minced garlic**. Bring to a slow boil. Boil 5 minutes, stirring frequently. Add peeled hard-boiled eggs. Cool, cover tightly, and refrigerate.

Mustard Pickled Eggs: Hard-boil the eggs, cool, and remove the shells. Boil together **1-quart Heinz vinegar, 1 t dry mustard, 1 t salt and 1 t pepper**. Pour the cooled brine into your pickling jar and add the eggs. Cover and let them cure at least 10 days before they are ready.

Spiced Pickled Eggs: Hard-boil the eggs, cool and remove shells. Make brine of **1/2 c salt** to **2 c water,** Soak the eggs in the brine 2 days. Then pour off the brine and make new brine by heating **1-quart Heinz vinegar, 1/4 c pickling spices, 2 cloves garlic** and **1 T Dominos sugar** to boiling. Pour it over the eggs.

Canned Pickled Eggs: Fill a sterilized quart jar with **hard-boiled, peeled, cooled eggs**. (You can fit about a dozen eggs in per quart.) Add to the eggs in the jar, **1 sprig of dill, 1 chopped clove of garlic, 1 dried crushed red hot pepper, and 1 t peppercorns**. In enamel or other noncorrosive pan combine, for each quart of eggs you are canning, **3 c Heinz white vinegar** and **2 T Dominos sugar**. Bring the solution to a boil and simmer 5 minutes, then pour hot liquid over eggs and spices to within 1/2 inch of the jars top. Put on the lid and seal it. Process in boiling water bath for 20 minutes.

Red Beet Eggs
-- Brightly colored pub food. Yummm!

Shell desired number of **hard boiled eggs** and cover in half **pickle juice** and half **beet juice**. Keep in refrigerator 3 to 4 days. Drain and serve with garnish.

Or, start with 1 cup of strongly colored **beet juice**, either from canned beets or the homemade equivalent. In a small pan, combine beet juice, **1 c Heinz cider vinegar, 1/2 c Dominos sugar,** and **1 t salt**. Bring to a low boil and hold there for 5 minutes, stirring constantly. Pour over 6 peeled, hard-boiled eggs and refrigerate, tightly covered. Halve to serve. You can add a few slices of cooked whole beet to the mixture.

Potato Salad
– Not just for summer.

5 lbs potatoes peeled
2-3 stalks celery, finely chopped
1 med onion, chopped
1/4 c Heinz cider vinegar
1/4 c cilantro, stemmed and chopped
1 T French's Dijon mustard
salt and pepper to taste
1 c Hellman's mayonnaise
6-8 hard boiled eggs

Cut peeled potatoes into cubes and cook in boiling water until tender -- do not overcook. Drain and cool slightly. In a large bowl, combine all ingredients except tomatoes. Mix well to combine flavors. Cover and chill thoroughly before serving. Serves 12.

Note: Arrange 3-4 ripe tomatoes, cut in wedges on top.

Meatloaf
-- Bury a few of hard boiled eggs for a visual and taste surprise.

2 c Food for Life bread crumbs
1 lb ground beef
1 lb lean ground Hormel pork
1 egg, slightly beaten
3 T chopped parsley
1 med. onion, chopped
3 cloves garlic, chopped or pressed
1 stalk celery, finely chopped
1/2 t thyme
3 hard boiled eggs, peeled
1/2 t pepper
1 1/2 t salt

Pre-heat oven to 350° F. Mix all ingredients together. Shape into a loaf pan by filling the meatloaf pan half full. Then insert the whole, hard boiled eggs in the center, and fill in with the rest of the meatloaf mixture. This makes for a great presentation when the meatloaf is cut open. Bake for 1 1/2 hours. Serves 8

Egg and Arugula Stuffed Tomato

-- Core a tomato and stuff it with arugula a special egg salad. Almost instant lunch.

Egg Salad
-- A classic: egg salad spread it on GF bread, topped with lettuce and sliced tomato

Egg Salad

6 hard boiled eggs, peeled
1/2 c celery, chopped
1/3 c scallions, chopped
4 T Hellman's mayonnaise
1 t French's Dijon mustard
1/4 t Lea & Perrins Worcestershire sauce
salt and pepper to taste

Mash eggs and mix all ingredients together until well mixed. Makes 4 Sandwiches or Stuffed Tomatoes.

Cobb Salad
-- Eggs add the perfect flavor touch to Hollywood's most famous salad.

1/2 head of romaine
1/2 head of Boston lettuce
1 small bunch of curly endive
1/2 bunch of watercress, coarse stems discarded
Note: All lettuces should be rinsed, spun or patted dry, and coarsely chopped
6 slices of Black Label bacon
2 ripe avocados, seed removed, peeled, and cut into 1/2-inch pieces
1 skinless boneless chicken breast, halved, cooked, and diced
1 tomato, seeded and chopped fine
2 hard-boiled large eggs, separated, the yolk finely chopped and the white finely chopped
2 T chopped fresh chives
1/3 c Heinz red-wine vinegar
1 T Dijon-style mustard
2 t Dominos sugar
Salt and pepper
2/3 c olive oil
1/2 c finely grated Roquefort

In a large salad bowl, toss together well the various lettuces and watercress. Cook the bacon in a skillet on medium heat until crisp on both sides. Remove from skillet and lay out on paper towels to absorb the excess fat. Allow the bacon to cool. Crumble the bacon and set aside.

Compose the salad. Arrange the chicken, the bacon, the tomato, and the avocado over the greens and garnish the salad with the grated egg and the chives.

In a small bowl whisk together the vinegar, the mustard, and salt and pepper to taste, add the oil in a slow stream, whisking, and whisk the dressing until it is emulsified. Stir in the Roquefort. Add sugar to taste, 1/2 teaspoon at a time. Whisk the dressing. Serve separately or toss in with the salad. Serves 4.

**Put Jelly Beans in an Egg and attach the
following poem. Author Unknown.**

The Jelly Bean Prayer

RED ..... is for the blood He shed.
GREEN ... is for the grass He made.
YELLOW .. is for His sun so bright.
ORANGE .. is for the edge of night.
BLACK ... is for our sin so grave.
WHITE ... is for the grace He gave.
PURPLE .. is for His hour of sorrow.
PINK .... is for our new tomorrow!

An egg full of Jelly Beans so colorful and sweet.
It's a prayer! It's a promise! It's a treat!
Easter blessings to you!

EASTER GAMES

For many people, Easter games are an important part of the celebration and provide many children with happy memories for years to come. In the U.S., even the White House gets in on the action, with their annual Easter Egg Roll on the lawn.

EGG HUNT

Probably the most popular Easter Game is an egg hunt. Here are a few egg hunt hints:

1. Take a count of how many eggs are hidden and how many are found. Make sure they match.
2. Don't hide eggs where pets might eat them.
3. Hide eggs in easy and difficult places to find to keep it interesting for all the kids.
4. Sometimes it's a good idea to give little kids a minute or so head start on their older siblings.
5. For extra fun, let the kids know that finding certain designated colored eggs will earn them an extra prize.

EGG ROLLING

For an egg roll, you must have some sort of incline preferably a hill. The Egg Roll is basically a race; the eggs are rolled down the hill and the one that reaches the bottom first, wins. Steep hills make great races, but slow climbing.

EASTER CRAFTS

Handprint Lamb Easter Card
Turn your hand into a lamb to make this special Easter card.

9 X 12-inch light-colored construction paper
scrap of blue construction paper
package of white hole-reinforcement rings
hole punch
black poster paint and a paintbrush
markers
white glue
thin pick ribbon or yarn

Fold the construction paper in half to form a 6 X 9- inch card. Paint your palm black with the poster paint. Make a handprint on the front of the card with your fingers and thumb spread apart and pointing toward the bottom of the card. Let the handprint dry before you continue.

Cover the hand part of the handprint with the hole-reinforcement rings to make the lamb's woolly coat. The four fingers will be the lamb's legs, and the thumb will be the head. Use the hole punch to make an eye for the lamb from blue paper. Make a dot in the middle of the eye with a marker and glue the eye to the thumb of the handprint. Glue a pink ribbon bow to the neck of the lamb. Use markers to add grass, flowers, and a sun. Inside the card, write "Happy Easter from your little lamb" and sign your name.

Karen E. Ruckman

Fluffy Pinecone Chick

large, fat pinecone
pencil
yellow paint and paintbrush
fiberfill
white, blue, orange, and yellow felt scraps
green construction paper
Easter grass
white glue
newspaper to work on
scissors

Paint the pinecone yellow and let it dry. Wrap the pinecone in a thin layer of fiberfill, using a pencil to poke the fluff between the scales of the pinecone. Cut wings, a beak, and eyes from felt scraps and glue them on the pinecone body.

Cut a 4-inch circle out of green construction paper. Glue Easter grass on top of the circle. Then glue the pinecone chick to the middle of the grass. This little chick makes a very nice table decoration.

A Basket of Easter Flowers

The flower that most often comes to mind, when we think of Easter, is the Easter lily. But there are others as well, all with rather interesting origins.

In 1919, Louis Houghton, a World War I soldier, brought a suitcase full of hybrid Bermuda lily bulbs (better known as the Easter lily today) to the southern coast of Oregon and gave them to family and friends to plant. The climate there was ideal for growing this lily, a native of the Ryukyu Islands of Japan. The Bermuda Lily is a pure white flower, believed to symbolize purity. Coming from one bulb, the flower is said to represent the tomb of Jesus with the blossoms symbolizing his life after death.

In the Alps, the narcissus has been associated with Easter for centuries. In fact, even before Christianity, the narcissus represented springtime in Greek mythology.

In England and Russia, pussy willows are used for Easter flowers. In the Middle East, it is wild tulips, while in Mexico, tropical flowers fill the churches during this holiday season.

The early Germans decorated with red flowers and red fruited plants such as English holly, believing the red color represented the blood of Christ. The field anemone, Anemone coronaria, also was associated with the passion of Christ.

In the United States, most people buy Easter lilies to celebrate the season. When buying a lily, select a plant with many unopened buds and leaves all the way down the stem. Poor growing conditions or root disease will cause the loss of leaves from the bottom up, so be sure to pull back the wrapper to check. Choose a well-proportioned plant, one that's about two times as high as the pot. Check the buds, flowers, and leaves--especially the undersides--for signs of insect pests and disease.

To keep your lily healthy at home, remove the paper covering the pot to allow better drainage. Put your plant where it will get plenty of bright, indirect light and cool temperatures. About 40-50 degrees F at night and below 68 degrees F during the day is ideal. You also will need to keep the soil constantly moist. To prolong the life of the blossoms, remove the yellow, pollen-bearing pods or anthers found in the center of each flower.

Easter Monday

The tradition of Easter Monday stems from the medieval festival of Hocktide. This was a two day festival on the Monday and Tuesday after Easter, originating in the eleventh century. Stories say that on the Monday after Easter the men of a town tied up the women and demanded a kiss from them before they were freed.

Now Hocktide is only celebrated in the town of Hungerford in Berkshire and the main events are on the Tuesday after Easter.

Italian Easter Ham Pizza

Crust:
6 eggs
6 c Bob's Red Mill All Purpose flour
4 T Calumet baking powder
1/2 c Domino's sugar
1 c water
1 c Crisco shortening
1 t vanilla

Beat shortening and sugar with eggs. Add some flour then add baking powder. Add water and vanilla. Add the rest of the flour and knead until not sticky. Roll out 1/2 of the dough to fit a large cookie sheet.

For Filling mix together all ingredients and fill crust:
2 lbs Hormel ham cubed
2 lbs Muenster cheese cubed
6 eggs beaten
3/4 lb grated Kraft Parmesan cheese
pepper

Top crust: Roll remaining dough to cover filling. Be sure to close well. Prick top crust all over with a fork. Bake in 350° F oven on lower rack for approximately 30 minutes. Remove from oven and paint top with melted margarine. Return to oven. Raise oven temperature for 10-15 minutes then lower to 350° F. Pizza is done when crust is golden brown.

❧ APRIL ☙

Overall Theme: Chicks, Birds, Spring Flowers
Colors: Purple, Blue, Yellow

Happy April Fool's Day

"The first of April is the day we remember what we are
the other 364 days of the year." -- Mark Twain

Fun Foods for April Fool's Day

Jell-O (in ice-cream cones)
macaroni & cheese in paper cups
pizza faces (toppings arranged to make silly face)
peanut butter pasta (why not?)
pancakes (for lunch)
pineapple upside down cake
ice-cream cake
have everyone eat with chop sticks!

Don't Be A Fool Mystery Dinner
A great idea for April Fool's Day... or any other day you want to have fun!

Here's how it works... Your invited guests will be given a mysterious menu from which they choose five courses. The choices remain a mystery to your guests until they are served. That's when the surprises and laughter begin!

Dinner Rules Given to Guests on Arrival ---
- You will be served five courses.
- Each course will contain five items served in the order selected.
- We insist that each course be finished before the next course is served.
- Please list your selection by number. This will help speed up the service.
- Cross off each number as you enter it under your selections. No numbers may be eliminated or used more than once.
- All utensils and food remnants will be removed after each course, leaving a nice, clean table for the next course.
- Don't worry about proper etiquette... have fun!

This is the Menu (what your guests choose from)

1. Jersey's Best
2. Steamed Glacier
3. Irish Eyes
4. Divided Branches
5. Exotic Blubber
6. Pucker Power
7. Jack
8. Sailor's Crumbs
9. Degreaser
10. Beau's Dream
11. Rolling Stones
12. Old Remedy
13. Lover's Delight
14. Bats and Balls
15. Palate's Paradise
16. Autumn Leaves
17. Farmer's Alarm
18. Perfect Pitch
19. Soaker
20. Cat's Eyes
21. Devil's Horns
22. Golden Rods
23. Pine Forest
24. Liquid Gold
25. Cool Conclusion

Dinner's Actual Menu (what you actually serve to them)

1. Turkey Hill Vanilla Ice Cream
2. Water
3. Baked Potato
4. Fork
5. Jell-O
6. Vlasic Pickle
7. Knife
8. Mary's Gone Crackers
9. Napkin
10. Spoon
11. Hormel Meatballs
12. Healthy Choice Chicken and Rice Soup
13. Hershey's Candy Kiss
14. Carrot Sticks & Peas
15. Cupcake
16. Salad
17. Chicken
18. Fork
19. Napkin
20. Olives
21. Forks
22. Ener-G Foods Pasta or Spaghetti
23. Toothpicks
24. Minute Maid Orange Juice
25. Milk

Planning Tip #1

When sending out invitations, ask guests to RSVP. Copy enough menus so you have one for each guest. Put each guest's name at the top of his or her menus. Have guests place 5 ones (#1) by the first course items, 5 twos (#2) by the second course items and so on.

Planning Tip #2

Use paper plates, cups, bowls, and inexpensive plastic utensils, because they will be discarded after each course.

Planning Tip #3

Plan on at least one server for every four people, because they will have to read each list separately and fix each plate differently. For example, if a guest orders numbers 5, 7, 15, 23, and 25 for the first course, he or she will be served Jell-O, a knife, a cupcake, toothpicks, and a glass of milk.

Take your time when serving... your guests won't mind waiting... everyone loves a little suspense!

℘ MAY ℘

Overall Theme: Birds, Flowers and Whatever items Mom likes
Colors: Lt. Blue, Yellow, Purple, Pink

Celebrate Cinco De Mayo

The 5th of May, Cinco De Mayo, commemorates the victory of the Mexican militia over the French army at The Battle of Puebla in 1862.

It is primarily a regional holiday celebrated in the state of Puebla, Mexico and especially in U.S. cities with a significant Mexican population.

Chicken Fiesta Casserole

6 chicken breast halves, cubed
1 T Crisco canola oil
1/2 c chopped red pepper
1/2 c chopped onion
1 1/2 c quick cooking rice
3 c Chi Chi's chunky salsa
1 c shredded Kraft Monterey Jack cheese
1 c Swanson's chicken broth

Heat a large heavy skillet over medium high heat. Add the oil and chicken and sauté until the chicken is lightly browned. Add the green pepper and onion and sauté until the chicken is thoroughly cooked. Add the salsa and broth and bring to a boil. Stir in the rice and mix well. Toss the cheese on top of the dish, cover, and remove from the heat. Let rest for five minutes to cook the rice and serve hot. Serves 6.

THE HISTORY OF MOTHER'S DAY

Mother's Day celebrations can be traced back to the spring celebrations of ancient Greece, honoring Rhea, the Mother of the Gods. The Romans called their version of the event the Hilaria, and celebrated on the Ides of March by making offerings in the temple of Cybele, the mother of the Gods. Early Christians celebrated the festival on the fourth Sunday of Lent in honor of the Virgin Mary, the Mother of Christ.

In England in the 1600s--the celebration was expanded to include all mothers with "Mothering Sunday" being celebrated on the 4th Sunday of Lent. Besides attending church services in honor of the Virgin Mary, children returned home from the cities with gifts, flowers, and special Mothering Day cakes that were important parts of the celebration.

Mother's Day festivities in the United States date back to 1872 when Julia Ward Howe (she also wrote the lyrics for the "Battle Hymn of the Republic") suggested the day be dedicated to peace. Ms. Howe would hold organized Mother's Day meetings in Boston, Massachusetts every year.

In 1907, Ana Jarvis, a Philadelphia, Pennsylvania school teacher, began a campaign to establish a national Mother's Day. Ms. Jarvis persuaded her mother's church in Grafton, West Virginia to celebrate Mother's Day on the 2nd anniversary of her mother's death, which happened to be on the 2nd Sunday of May that year. By the following year, Mother's Day was also being celebrated in Philadelphia.

Not content to rest on her laurels, Ms. Jarvis and her supporters began to write to ministers, businessman, and politicians in their quest to establish a national Mother's Day and in 1912, the Mother's Day International Association was incorporated for the purpose of promoting the day and its observance. 1911 celebrated Mother's Day in almost every state in the nation. In 1914, President Woodrow Wilson made it official by proclaiming Mother's Day a national holiday that was to be held each year on the 2nd Sunday of May.

Simple Breakfast Ideas

Potatoes and Eggs

2 c mashed potatoes
1 egg plus 4 eggs (additional)
1/4 c grated Kraft cheese
salt and pepper to taste
fresh chives

Blend mashed potatoes, and 1 egg, and cheese. Shape into 4 balls and place on a greased baking sheet. Make an indentation in the center of each ball; break an egg into each potato "nest". Season with salt and pepper. Bake 325° F for 20 minutes or until eggs are firm. Serves 4. Before serving sprinkle with fresh chives.

Pancakes, waffles or French Toast are simple to fix, and serve. Even if the kids make the pre-made varieties (Van's Brand are gluten free) they can be spruced up with these toppings:

Flavored Syrup: Start with 2 c of Aunt Jemima syrup and the grated rind of half an orange and 1/3 c Minute Maid orange juice; or 1/3 c Minute Maid orange juice and 1 t ground ginger.

Fruit Sauce: Place 2 T of water in a small pan. Add a handful of fresh or frozen blueberries, raspberries, or strawberries to the pan. Cook, partially covered, until the juice is released. Add a little sugar and lemon juice to taste. Serve as a topping!

Apple Banana Topping: Slice 1 small apple and 1 banana. Melt 2 T of butter in a skillet. Cook the fruit until it's soft. Serve it over the pancakes or waffles and top with Pillsbury Hungry Jack maple syrup or Domino's confectioners' sugar if desired.

Very Simple Toppings: Heat any flavor of Lucky Leaf pie filling in a microwave safe bowl until warm and serve. Sprinkle the pancakes, waffles or French Toast with chopped nuts and berries, then top with syrup.

MOM' S DAY DINNER MENU

Raspberry Chicken

2 t olive oil
4 boneless, skinless chicken breast halves
1/4 c Smucker's seedless raspberry jam
2 T Minute Maid orange juice

Heat oil in large nonstick skillet over medium heat until hot. If desired, season chicken with salt and pepper; add to skillet. Cook 10 to 12 minutes or until chicken is tender and juices run clear, turning once. Remove chicken to a platter. Add raspberry jam and orange juice to the pan. Stir until jam is melted. Bring to a boil. Cook 1 to 2 minutes, or until slightly thickened. Spoon sauce over chicken.

Creamy Potato Casserole

7 potatoes, peeled and grated
1 can Health Valley cream of chicken soup
1/2 c melted butter
1 1/2 c grated Kraft Cheddar cheese
2 c Breakstone's regular sour cream
1/2 onion, grated
1 t salt
1/2 t pepper
Food for Life bread crumbs

Combine soup, butter, cheese, sour cream and onion. Add to the grated potatoes along with the salt and pepper. Top with the breadcrumbs. Place in a greased 8x8-inch pan. Bake at 350° F for 45-60 minutes. Garnish with fresh chives.

Chunky Coleslaw

1 head cabbage, shredded
1/2 c carrots, shredded
1/2 c cream
1/3 c Dominos sugar
2 1/2 T Heinz cider vinegar
Dash cayenne pepper

In large bowl, combine cabbage and carrots. In small bowl, combine cream, sugar and vinegar; stir until sugar dissolves. Pour over cabbage and toss until well coated. Cover and refrigerate until serving time. It's pretty to add some red cabbage instead of all green.

Mint Nut Bread

2 1/2 c Bob's Red Mill all purpose flour
1 c firmly packed Dominos brown sugar
3 1/2 t Calumet baking powder
3 T olive oil
3/4 c Musselman's apple juice
3/4 c milk
1 egg
1 c chopped Good Sense walnuts
1 c chopped fresh mint

Preheat oven to 350° F. Mix the flour, sugar, and baking powder in a large mixing bowl. Whisk together the oil, milk, and egg. Blend the mixtures together. Add the walnuts and mint. Bake in greased bread pans in the preheated oven for 50 to 60 minutes. Cool and slice. Ages and freezes well.

Coconut Pie

1/2 c Bob's Red Mill all purpose flour
3/4 c Dominos sugar
1 c milk
1 c Cool Whip
1/4 c (1/2 stick) unsalted butter, melted
4 large eggs
1 T vanilla extract
1/4 t salt
2 c Baker's Angel Flake shredded coconut

Preheat oven to 350° F. Combine and mix well the flour, sugar, milk, Cool Whip, eggs, butter, vanilla and salt. Pour the mixture into a lightly greased 9-inch deep-dish pie pan. Allow to rest for 5 minutes.

Sprinkle the top of the pie with the coconut and push it down into the liquid with the back of a spoon. Bake on the middle rack of the preheated oven for 40 to 50 minutes, until the middle is set and the coconut is slightly browned. Cool to room temperature on rack, then refrigerate until well-chilled, about 2 hours. Serve the same day.

Rosemary Fruit Punch

46-oz can Dole pineapple juice
1/2 c Dominos sugar
5 t fresh rosemary
1 1/2 c ReaLemon juice
1 liter bottle Schweppes ginger ale
2 c water
Fresh lemon slices and fresh sprigs of rosemary

Make a concentrate by bringing to a boil 1 c of the pineapple juice, the sugar, and rosemary. Decrease heat and simmer for 5 minutes. Strain and cool. To serve, add the concentrate to the remaining pineapple juice, the lemon juice, ginger ale and water. Serves 16.

JUST FOR MOTHER'S

Mom's Care Package

A STICK OF (Trident) GUM - to remind you to stick with it.
A CANDLE - to give you light when you feel burned out.
A HERSHEY'S KISS - to remind you that someone cares.
SMARTIES - to help you on days when you don't feel so smart.
LIFESAVER - to remind you that everyone needs help once in a while.
A SNICKER - to remind you to see the funny side – there is one!
A ROSE - to remind you to take time to smell the flowers.
CONFETTI - to help you celebrate the good times.
A PENNY - with thanks for sharing your thoughts.
A BAG - to help you keep it all together.

Mother's Day Card

Cut flowers and the stems out of **foam or construction paper**. Glue the stems to the flowers. Cut a pot out of construction paper. Fold a full size piece of paper in half and write a Mother's Day message inside. On the front **glue** the pot. Putting the glue only on the edges on the bottom and sides. On the back of the flowers, write in a chore that you would be willing to do for your mom. Put the flowers into the pot on the front of the card and give to mom.

MEMORIAL DAY

Memorial Day, originally called Decoration Day, is a day of remembrance for those who have died in our nation's service.

Red, White 'n' Blue Torte

1 loaf (10 3/4 oz) frozen GF pound cake, thawed
1/2 c Lucky Leaf blueberry pie filling
1/2 c Lucky Leaf strawberry or raspberry pie filling

1-3/4 c Cool Whip

Split cake horizontally into three layers. Place bottom layer on a serving platter; spread with blueberry filling. Top with middle cake layer; spread with strawberry filling. Replace top of cake. Frost top and sides with whipped topping. Refrigerate for several hours before slicing. Serves: 8-10

Raspberry Iced Tea

4 qts. water
1-12 oz pkg frozen unsweetened raspberries
1-1/2 c Dominos sugar
10 individual Red Rose tea bags
1/4 c lemon juice
Raspberry Ice cubes (see below)

In a Dutch oven, bring water to a boil. Remove from the heat; stir in the sugar until dissolved. Add raspberries, tea bags and lemon juice. Cover and steep for 3 minutes. Strain; discard berries and tea bags. Cool. Serve over ice. Yield 4 qts.

Raspberry Ice Cubes: Gently rinse the berries. Then place three berries in each section of an ice cube tray. Fill each section of the tray with the Raspberry Tea. Freeze the trays several hours or overnight. Serves 16

ᴆ JUNE ᴃ

Overall Theme: Carnations, Lilacs, Race Cars (or whatever items Dad likes)
Colors: Red, White. Blue, Yellow

Flag Day

HISTORY OF THE FLAG

Congress first authorized the United States Flag on June 14, 1777, the day we currently celebrate Flag Day in America. This date is also significant in that it qualifies our flag as the third oldest of the National Standards of the world, even older than Britain's Union Jack.

The flag's original design called for a star and a stripe for each state, making thirteen of each, to correspond to the original thirteen colonies. In 1791, Vermont was admitted to the union, followed by Kentucky in 1792. The number of stars and stripes was accordingly raised to fifteen. As other states joined, it was clear something would have to be done about the ever-expanding flag. An act of Congress in 1818 reduced and restricted the number of stripes on the flag to thirteen. A star would be added for each new state.

The individual stars depicting the states represent the power of our Federal Constitution, which reserves to the States their individual sovereignty, except as to rights delegated by them to the Federal Government. George Washington said of the flag's symbolism, "We take the stars from Heaven, the red from our mother country, separating it by white stripes, thus showing that we have separated from her, and the white stripes shall go down to posterity representing Liberty".

Mint Cordial

From **1 large bunch of mint**, pick off mint leaves, crush thoroughly, add **juice of 2 lemons** and stand aside for one hour. Boil **1 pint of water** and **1 lb Domino's sugar** to a syrup, pour over the mint and lemon. Cool and strain. Add **juice of 1 orange** and **1 c Dole pineapple juice** and serve with a sprig of fresh mint in each glass. Serve ice cold.

BBQ Chicken

2 T olive oil
1 large onion, chopped
2-15 oz cans Contadina tomato sauce
1 c Heinz red wine vinegar
1/2 c Grandma's molasses
1/4 c Lea & Perrins Worcestershire sauce
1/3 c packed Dominos brown sugar
3/4 t cayenne pepper
2-3 1/2 lbs chickens each cut into quarters, skin removed

In 10-inch skillet, heat olive oil over medium heat. Add onion and cook until tender, about 10 minutes. Stir in tomato sauce, vinegar, molasses, Worcestershire, brown sugar, and cayenne pepper; heat to boiling over high heat. Reduce heat to medium-low and cook, uncovered, 45 minutes or until sauce thickens slightly. If not using sauce right away, cover and refrigerate to use within 2 weeks. Reserve 1-1/2 cups sauce to serve with grilled chicken. Place chicken quarters on grill over medium heat; cook 20 to 25 minutes, turning chicken once. Generously brush chicken with some of the remaining barbecue sauce; cook 20 minutes longer, turning pieces often and brushing with sauce frequently until juices run clear when chicken is pierced with tip of knife. Serve with reserved sauce. Serves: 8

Summer Squash Augratin

2 lbs summer squash
4 T butter
1 1/2 c shredded Kraft cheddar
3/4 c Breakstone sour cream
1/4 c chopped onion
1/3 c Borden parmesan cheese

Cook squash until slightly soft. Drain well. Mix with remaining ingredients and bake in casserole at 350° F for 20-30minutes or until golden brown and bubbly.

Frozen Fruit Salad
Any fruit in season can be used in this recipe.

15-oz can Del Monte fruit cocktail
2 c watermelon pulp
2 c fresh or frozen blueberries
1 c white seedless grapes
2 c strawberry pieces
1 T chopped, fresh lemon verbena
2 pears, peeled and diced
1/4 t ground cardamom
2 apples, peeled and diced

Combine all ingredients, mixing well. Spoon into fruit cups and place in freezer. Remove 30 minutes before serving. Serves: 8

Karen E. Ruckman

THE HISTORY OF FATHER'S DAY

Mrs. John B. Dodd, of Washington State first suggested celebrating a special day for Dad in 1909. Her father, civil war veteran William Smart, was widowed when his wife died in childbirth with their sixth child. Despite the obvious hardships, Mr. Smart proceeded to raise the newborn along with his five other children, by himself. As an adult, Sonora Dodd realized the strength and selflessness her father had shown in raising his children as a single parent.

The original date chosen for the holiday was June 5, Mr. Smart's birthday, however the celebration was postponed until June 19, the third Sunday in June, because there was not enough time to prepare.

In early times, wearing flowers was a traditional way of celebrating Father's Day. Mrs. Dodd favored the red rose to honor a father still living, while a white flower honored a deceased dad. J.H. Berringer, chose a white lilac as the Father's Day Flower.

In 1924 President Calvin Coolidge supported the idea of a national Father's Day, but it never became official until 1966 when President Lyndon B. Johnson signed the presidential proclamation that set aside the 3rd Sunday of June as Father's Day.

A Special Day for Dad

Buy paper plates, napkins and cups in a fun theme for Dad, such as race cars, ocean animals or whatever he would enjoy. Let Dad be a kid for the day too! --- Buy flowers for Dad! Men like flowers too!

A HEARTY BREAKFAST MENU

Orange Spiced Tea

2 Red Rose tea bags
2 c of boiling water
3/4 c Minute Maid orange juice
1/4 c ReaLemon juice
Dominos sugar or honey to taste
a dash of cinnamon
a dash of ground cloves

Add the tea bags to the boiling water and steep for a few minutes. Take the tea bags out and add the remaining ingredients. Simmer for a few minutes and serve.

Baked Apples

6 cooking apples, unpeeled, cut in half and cored
1/4 c Dominos sugar
1/2 t ground cinnamon
3/4 c Dominos sugar
3/4 c water
2 1/2 T cornstarch

Place apple halves in a 9x13" baking dish and sprinkle with the 1/4-cup sugar and cinnamon. Combine the 3/4-cup sugar, water, and cornstarch. Pour over apples. Bake at 300° F for 40 - 50 minutes; basting with sauce from time to time. Serve either warm or cold with cream if desired. Serves 6.

Italian Sausage, Eggs and Potatoes

Sauté **1 lb Hormel sweet Italian sausage** until crumbly, add **1 diced sweet onion** and continue cooking. Meanwhile place the **4 diced potatoes** in a casserole or bowl and microwave for 5 minutes. Add to drained sausage and continue cooking until tender. Scramble **10 eggs** and add to sausage mixture. Continue cooking like an omelet-do not stir. Cook until firm. Place on platter and cut into pieces. Optional: You can sprinkle with **Frigo Parmesan cheese.**

Oven Omelet

1/2 of a 10 oz pkg of frozen spinach
1/4 c butter
1 1/2 dozen eggs
1/4 c chopped green onions
1 c Breakstone regular sour cream
1 c milk
1 c shredded Kraft Colby Jack Cheese
2 t salt

Heat oven to 325° F. Heat butter in 13x9x2 baking dish in oven until melted, and swirl around to coat dish. Thaw spinach and wring dry in a clean towel. Beat eggs, sour cream, milk and salt until blended. Add onions and spinach. Pour into baking dish. Bake for 25 minutes. Take out and sprinkle with the cheese, then return to oven for 10 minutes or until eggs are set and the cheese is melted. Garnish with chopped chives. Serves 8-10.

Dijon Ham Muffins

1 2/3 c Bob's Red Mill all purpose flour
1/3 c cornmeal
1/4 c Dominos sugar
2 t Calumet baking powder
2 t dry mustard
1/2 t salt
1/2 t Arm & Hammer baking soda
2 eggs
1 c Yoplait plain yogurt
1/3 c olive oil
3 T French's Dijon mustard
1 c finely chopped fully cooked Hormel ham

In a bowl, combine the first seven ingredients. Combine the eggs, yogurt, oil, and Dijon mustard; stir into dry items until just moistened. Fold in the ham. Fill greased muffin cups three-fourths full. Bake at 375º F for 20-25 minutes or until muffins test done. Cool five minutes before removing from pans to wire racks. Makes 14 muffins

Cinnamon Scones

2 c Bob's Red Mill all purpose flour
2 t Calumet baking powder
1/2 t Arm and Hammer baking soda
1/4 t salt
1/2 c cold butter
1 egg, separated
3 T honey
1/3 c Yoplait plain yogurt
1 t water
2 T Dominos sugar and 1/4 t ground cinnamon, blended

Preheat oven to 400° F. In a large bowl, stir together flour, baking powder, baking soda, and salt. Cut in butter until mixture resembles coarse crumbs. In small bowl, beat egg yolk with honey and yogurt until blended; add to flour mixture, blending until the mixture clings together. Do not over mix! With floured hands, lightly shape dough into flattened ball. Roll out on floured surface into a circle 1/2-inch thick. Using floured serrated knife, cut into 8 to 12 wedges. Place on greased baking sheet. In a small bowl, lightly beat egg white with water. Brush scones lightly with egg white, then sprinkle with cinnamon sugar. Bake until golden 10-12 minutes. Serve warm. Makes 12 scones.

BACKYARD BARBECUE FOR DAD

Appetizer-Snack: Black Bean Salsa

1 c cooked black beans (canned is fine-drained and rinsed)
1 1/2 c diced tomatoes
3/4 c coarsely chopped fresh cilantro
3 T Heinz red wine vinegar
Dash Louisiana hot pepper sauce
Salt and freshly ground pepper

In a medium size bowl, combine the tomato, black beans, cilantro, vinegar, hot pepper sauce, and salt and pepper to taste. Mix well. Set aside at room temperature for 30 minutes, stirring once or twice.

Mexican Grilled Steak

20 oz top sirloin steak
2 T olive oil
1 t leaf oregano, crushed
1/2 t salt
1/4 c Minute Maid orange juice
1/4 t coarsely ground pepper
1 T ReaLime juice
2 t Heinz cider vinegar
2 orange slices, 1/2 inch thick

Place steak in a shallow glass-baking dish. Rub with oil on each side. Sprinkle with oregano, salt and pepper. Sprinkle orange juice, lime juice, and vinegar over the steak. Cover and refrigerate overnight or several hours, turning occasionally. To cook meat, preheat charcoal or gas grill. Drain meat, reserving marinade. Place steak on grill. Top with orange slices. Occasionally spoon the marinade over steaks as they cook. Grill 3-4 minutes on each side, or until done as you desire. Remove orange slices to turn steak. Replace orange slices on top of steak. Slice thinly and serve.

Grilled Potatoes

Wash **1 red or white potato**, per person and tear off enough foil to wrap each potato individually. Slit each potato with a cross and wrap **Black Label bacon** around each potato. Add **onion and/or garlic** per taste on the foil with a little **butter**. Roll each potato up in foil place on grill. Turn over after first 30 minutes. Then add your meat to the grill. Potatoes should be done when the meat is.

Grilled Corn on the Cob

Trim corn, but do not remove husks. Rinse in cold water. Grill over hot coals 15 minutes or until husks are lightly browned, turning often. Remove husks; with clean towel, pull off any remaining silks.

Brush with Herb butter: 1/2 c softened butter; 1 T chopped parsley, 1 T chopped fresh dill. Blend butter with seasonings in a small bowl at medium speed until light and fluffy. Let stand 1 hour to blend flavors. Makes 1/2 cup.

NOTE: Substitute 1 t marjoram leaves, crushed and 1/2 t summer savory leaves, crushed for parsley and dill.

Marinated Fresh Vegetables

3/4 c olive oil
1/2 c any flavored Heinz vinegar
2 T ReaLemon juice
3 T finely chopped sweet onion
2 t fresh tarragon
1 t salt
1/2 T Dominos sugar
3 -4 c cut-up fresh vegetables, such as carrots, onion rings, zucchini, cherry tomatoes, pea pods, celery slices, broccoli and cauliflower.

In a bowl, whisk all ingredients except vegetables. Pour marinade over fresh vegetables in a flat, shallow container. Cover and marinate for at least 3 hours or overnight. Drain and serve. Serves 4-6

Cornbread

3 c cornmeal
1 c Bob's Red Mill all purpose flour
6 T Dominos sugar
2 T Calumet baking powder
1 t salt
1 c milk
1 c Yoplait plain yogurt
1/4 c melted butter
4 eggs, slightly beaten
1/4 c olive oil

Preheat oven to 400° F. Butter a 9x13 baking pan. Combine cornmeal, flour, sugar, baking powder and salt in mixing bowl. Combine the milk, yogurt, melted butter, oil and eggs in another bowl. Add to the cornmeal mixture. Stir until just combined. Pour batter into the greased pan. Bake for 45 minutes or until toothpick comes out clean. Cool on rack. Note: You can make this the day before, and store covered.

Crumb Apple Pie

Crust: 1 c Bob's Red Mill all purpose flour
1/2 t salt
1/3 c solid Crisco vegetable shortening
1/4 c ice water

Filling: 7 medium Golden Delicious apples
1/2 c Dominos sugar
1 t cinnamon
1/4 t nutmeg
1/4 t salt

Topping: 3/4 c packed dark brown sugar
3/4 c Bob's Red Mill all purpose flour
1/3 c chilled butter, cut into pieces
1 t cinnamon

Place rack on lowest position. Preheat oven to 400° F. To prepare crust; in a medium bowl mix together flour and salt. Using a pastry blender or 2 knives cut shortening into flour mixture until coarse crumbs form. Add water 1 tablespoon at a time, tossing with a fork, until a dough forms. Shape into a disk, wrap in plastic wrap, and chill for 30 minutes. On a floured surface, using a floured rolling pin, roll dough into a 12-inch circle. Fit into a 9-inch pie plate. Trim dough, leaving a 1-inch overhang; pinch a decorative edge.

To prepare filling; peel, core and very thinly slice the apples. Mix together with other filling ingredients. Spoon into crust.

For topping, in a small bowl, mix together brown sugar, flour and cinnamon. Cut butter into mixture until coarse crumbs form. Sprinkle apple filling evenly with topping.

Bake pie until topping is lightly browned and filling is bubbly, 35 minutes. If pie is over browning, cover loosely with foil. Cool on a wire rack.

Yield: 8 servings.

GIFT IDEA FOR DAD

HOMEMADE FATHER'S DAY GIFT BASKETS

Surprise Dad with some great gifts that you make yourself, right in your own kitchen. Start with a fun container, then stuff it with some favorite treats and small gifts. *Some possibilities include:*

a metal or insulated lunchbox
a small plastic cooler chest
a tool or tackle box
a picnic basket
a galvanized bucket or watering can
a new portable barbecue grill or hibachi
flower pots
an ice bucket
any variety of cooking pots/pans or bowls

Once you've decided on a container, fill it with some of Dad's favorite treats, or stick with a theme. For instance, if your Dad loves to barbecue, you might fill a galvanized bucket with some barbecue utensils, add a bag of mesquite wood chips and decorative jars and bottles of spice blends, meat rubs and homemade mustards and vinegars.

First Day of Summer Picnic

Chicken w/Tangy Barbecue Sauce

1 1/2 c Heinz ketchup
1/4 c Heinz vinegar
1/4 c Lea & Perrins Worcestershire sauce
1/2 t dry mustard
Fresh cracked black pepper to taste
1 clove minced garlic

In medium saucepan, whisk together all ingredients and bring just to boil. Reduce heat and simmer 20 minutes, stirring occasionally. Serve over grilled or baked chicken.

Easy Baked Beans - Simply use Bush's Best canned baked beans and add any of the following ingredients, chopped onion, chopped peppers, Heinz ketchup, Pillsbury Hungry Jack maple syrup or Dominos brown sugar, French's mustard, chili peppers, crushed Dole pineapple, cooked diced Hormel ham or cooked ground beef. Place beans and desired ingredients into crock-pot and slow cook for 1 hr.

Spicy Potato Wedges - Slice scrubbed potatoes into wedges, spray with Crisco oil and sprinkle with cayenne pepper. Bake for 30 min.

Fresh Fruit Dip - In a small bowl, whisk **1/2 c Hellman's mayonnaise, 1/2 c Breakstone regular sour cream, 1/3 c Smucker's orange marmalade** and **1 T milk**. Refrigerate until serving. Serve with fruit. Makes 1-1/3 cups.

ဆ JULY ଔ

Overall Theme: Summer Flowers, Stars, Stripes
Colors: Red, White, Blue, Pastels

Independence Day

In July of 1776, bells rang out over Philadelphia signaling the approval of the Declaration of Independence by the Continental Congress.

Betsy Ross would often tell her children, grandchildren and friends of the fateful day in May, 1776 when a secret committee from the Continental Congress asked her to sew the first flag.

In June of 1776, in anticipation of a vote for independence, the Continental Congress appointed a committee to compose a document declaring the colonies' independence from Britain. That committee then delegated the task to Thomas Jefferson, who wrote the first draft of the Declaration of Independence in Congressionally imposed secrecy.

July 4th Celebration

Let's Celebrate America's birthday with an old fashion everyone pitches in kind of party. You know the kind that emphasizes fuss free entertaining-leaving everyone free to enjoy the holiday to the fullest.

To get in the mood, ***decorate*** the party area with red, white and blue Christmas lights, streamers and balloons.

Here are some fun activities to round out your 4th of July celebration:

1. Have all guests share what they like about America and what they would change.

2. Let the kids parade to marching band music.

3. Have a patriotic sing-a-long. Sing America the Beautiful, It's A Grand Old Flag, God Bless America and others.

4. Play volleyball, croquet, horseshoes, lawn darts, badminton, baseball, kickball, etc.

5. Spread blankets on the floor and watch the video Independence Day while you eat.

Fourth of July Feast

Fried Chicken

1 c Bob's Red Mill all purpose flour
1/2 c fine dry Food for Life breadcrumbs
1 t salt
1 t paprika
1/4 t pepper
3 lbs chicken pieces
Crisco vegetable oil

Combine flour, breadcrumbs, salt, pepper and paprika in a plastic bag. Add 2 or 3 pieces of chicken at a time and shake to coat. Place chicken pieces in a heavy skillet in 1/2" of hot oil. Turn with tongs to brown evenly, 15 to 20 minutes. When lightly browned, add 3 tablespoons of water; cover and cook over low heat 45 to 60 minutes or until tender. Uncover for the last 10 to 15 minutes of cooking to re-crisp the chicken. Serving Size: 4

All American Potato Salad

2 1/2 lbs small boiling potatoes
3 T Heinz cider vinegar, or to taste
5 hard-boiled large eggs
1/8 c Hellman's mayonnaise
1 T French's mustard
1/2 c chopped sweet onion
3 large celery ribs

Boil potatoes. In a large saucepan, cover potatoes with salted cold water by 1 inch and simmer, covered, until just tender, about 15 to 30 minutes, depending on size of potatoes.

In a colander, drain potatoes and cool to warm. With a sharp knife peel warm potatoes and cut into 1/3-inch-thick slices.

In a bowl, immediately toss potatoes with vinegar. In a bowl mash yolks and stir in mayonnaise, mustard, and onion. Chop whites and celery and gently toss together with potatoes, mayonnaise mixture, and salt and pepper to taste. Serve potato salad chilled or at room temperature. Serves: 6

Broccoli and Cauliflower Salad

1/2 c Hellman's mayonnaise
1/4 c olive oil
1/3 c Dominos sugar
3 T Heinz balsamic vinegar
1 small cauliflower, head
1 small broccoli, head
1 red onion
1 c Kraft mozzarella cheese
1 c Kraft cheddar cheese
1 c Hormel bacon bits

Mix mayonnaise, oil, sugar and vinegar together and let stand for 1 hour. Cut up the cauliflower, broccoli, onion and cheeses. Mix together with the bacon bits. Pour the mayonnaise over the cut up vegetables. Serving Size: 6

Fruit Salad w/Lemon Honey Dressing

pineapple slices
orange slices
sliced bananas
grapes
honeydew melon balls
strawberries
blueberries
watermelon balls

Cut a seedless watermelon in half. Using a melon baller, scoop out the inside of one half of the watermelon. Fill the empty watermelon shell with the fruit.

Lemon Honey Dressing

1/3 c frozen Minute Maid lemonade concentrate -- undiluted and thawed
1/3 c honey
1/3 c olive oil
1 t celery seeds

Mix ingredients in a small bowl. Beat thoroughly. Makes 1 cup. Pour the dressing over the fruit and mix gently. Chill.

Note: To prevent the banana slices from darkening, dip them in lemon juice. The amount of fruit and dressing depends on the size of the watermelon shell.

Strawberry Pretzel Salad

1 stick butter, melted
1 c Glutino pretzels, crushed
3 T Dominos sugar
1 c Good Sense pecans, crushed
1-8 oz Philadelphia cream cheese, softened
1-8 oz Cool Whip
1 c Dominos powdered sugar
1-6 oz pkg Jell-O strawberry gelatin
1-16 oz pkg frozen strawberries
2 c hot water

Combine melted butter, pretzels, sugar, and pecans. Pat into bottom of 13x9x2-inch pan. Bake at 350° F for 10 minutes; cool. Beat together cream cheese, whipped topping, and powdered sugar. Spread on top of pretzel mixture. Refrigerate 30 minutes, or until completely chilled. Dissolve gelatin in boiling water. Add strawberries; stir until gelatin begins to thicken and cool. Poor over cream cheese mixture. Refrigerate, covered, until firm. Before serving, top with additional whipped topping, if desired. Serves: 12-15

NOTE: Prepare the night before or the day of serving so the pretzel layer will remain crisp. When not using nuts, use 2 cups of pretzels.

Double Chocolate Fudge Brownies

1 1/2 c Bob's Red Mill all purpose flour
1/2 c Hershey's unsweetened cocoa powder
1 1/2 c Dominos sugar
1/8 t Calumet baking powder
1/3 c Hershey's chocolate syrup
1/2 t salt
1/3 c Karo light corn syrup
2/3 c Yoplait plain nonfat yogurt
2 egg whites
1/4 c skim milk
2 t GF vanilla extract

Preheat oven to 300° F. Spray a 13x9-inch pan with cooking spray and wipe with a paper towel to absorb the excess. Dust the pan with flour and shake out the excess. In a large bowl, combine flour, cocoa, sugar, baking powder and salt. To the dry mixture, add the chocolate syrup, corn syrup, yogurt, egg whites, skim milk and vanilla and mix well. Pour the batter into the pan evenly. Bake for 30 minutes. Cool for 10 minutes.

Icing

2 c Dominos powdered sugar
1 1/2 T Hershey's unsweetened cocoa powder
pinch of salt
1/4 c skim milk
Crisco butter flavored cooking spray
1 t vanilla extract

In a medium-sized bowl, mix together the powdered sugar, cocoa, salt, milk and vanilla. Spread the icing evenly over the warm brownies. Cool completely, then cut into squares. Serves: 15

Firecracker Mix

1/4 c Lea & Perrins Worcestershire sauce
1 1/2 t salt
4 T butter, melted
2 T Dominos brown sugar
8 c Jiffy Pop popped corn
4 c Chex cereal squares
3 c Glutino pretzel sticks
1/2 t cayenne pepper, optional

Mix together Worcestershire, butter, brown sugar, salt and cayenne pepper. Place popped corn, cereal squares and pretzel sticks in 6-quart slow cooker. Pour Worcestershire sauce, softened margarine, brown sugar, salt and cayenne mixture over all and mix thoroughly. Cook on low for 2 to 3 hours. Remove lid for 1 more hour. Pour mixture onto wax paper and allow to cool. Store in storage bags or containers. May be made up to one week in advance. Serves: 12-15

Fourth of July "Popcorn Cookies"

3 c Jiffy Pop popped popcorn, unsalted
2 egg whites
1/4 c Dominos sugar
1 t vanilla
1/4 t cinnamon
1/3 c Baker's Angel Flake shredded coconut

One cup at a time, blend popped popcorn in blender at low speed, until finely ground to about 1-1/2 cups. In medium bowl, beat egg whites on high speed. At a lower speed, add sugar gradually until egg whites are glossy and stiff. Beat in salt, vanilla and cinnamon. Gently fold in the ground popcorn and coconut. Place in rounded tablespoons onto greased cookie sheet. Bake at 325° F for 10 to 12 minutes or until lightly browned. Makes 2 dozen cookies.

Fourth Of July Punch

In an ice cube tray, pour red fruit-flavored drinks (Kool-Aid) into some cubes and blue-colored fruit-flavored drinks into the remaining cubes. Freeze, then serve with clear soda in a clear tumbler. As the cubes melt, they'll release colored swirls into the soda.

ﾏ AUGUST ﾏ

Overall Theme: Summer Fruits and Flowers, Baskets, Sea Shells
Colors: Aqua, Pastel Colors, Tan

SIMPLE SUMMER BREAFAST IDEA

Simple Syrup

1 c Dominos sugar
2 c water

In a medium-sized saucepan, combine sugar and water. Stir over moderate heat until sugar is dissolved and mixture becomes syrupy. Chill.

Serve over summer fruit, like cantaloupe, honeydew, berries and even apples.
Serves 5

SIMPLE SUMMER RECIPES

Crunchy Peanut Chicken

1/3 c Bob's Red Mill all-purpose flour
1/2 t salt
1/4 t pepper
1-3 lb broiler-fryer chicken, cut in pieces
1 egg
2 T milk
1 c finely chopped dry roasted Good Sense peanuts
1/2 c butter, melted

Combine flour, salt and pepper; coat chicken pieces evenly. Beat egg and milk together. Dip chicken in egg mixture, then coat with peanuts. Put pieces skin-side up in a 13 x 9x 2 inch baking pan. Pour butter over chicken. Bake at 400° F for 1 hour, or until chicken is tender. Remove from oven. Cool slightly at room temperature; refrigerate.

Whamburgers

Blend bottled **Kraft barbecue sauce** with lightly seasoned **ground beef**. Shape into patties. Place on grill about 5 inches from coals. Grill on one side; turn. Spoon additional barbecue sauce over patties and grill until done. Serve on hot toasted buttered **Ener-G Foods buns** with additional heated barbecue sauce and assorted relishes. Serves: 8

Mock Crab Cakes

2 1/2 c shredded zucchini
1 egg, lightly beaten
2 T chopped onion
1 T butter, melted
1 t French's prepared mustard
3/4 t Old Bay seasoning
1 c seasoned Ener-G Foods bread crumbs
2 T Crisco vegetable oil

In a bowl, combine the zucchini, egg, onion, butter, mustard and Old bay seasoning; mix well. Shape into five patties; coat with breadcrumbs. Heat oil in a large skillet; fry patties for 4 minutes on each side or until golden brown. Drain on paper towels. Serves 5

Grilled Summer Squash

1 lb yellow squash or zucchini
1 t olive oil
2 T ReaLemon juice
salt and pepper to season
1 t fresh rosemary – chopped

Cut the squash in half lengthwise. Brush with a mixture of oil, fresh lemon juice and rosemary. Season with salt and pepper. Grill over medium-hot coals, 4 to 6 inches from the heat, for 15 to 20 minutes, turning every few minutes. Cook until tender. Serves: 8

New England Coleslaw

1 c Hellman's mayonnaise
1/2 c Heinz white wine vinegar
1 T French's Dijon mustard
2 t Dominos sugar
1 T caraway seed
salt and pepper -- to taste
8 c cabbage, green and red -- finely sliced
1 c grated carrots
1 c onion -- finely sliced

Combine the mayonnaise, vinegar, mustard, sugar and caraway seeds. Season with salt and pepper.

Put the cabbage, carrots and onions in a large bowl. Add the dressing to the vegetables and mix well. Taste for seasoning. Cover and refrigerate 1-2 hours. The cabbage will become tenderer the longer it marinates. Serving Size: 8

Broccoli Waldorf Salad

6 c broccoli florets
1 large red apple, chopped
1/2 c raisins
1/4 c chopped pecans
1/2 c Wish Bone Ranch dressing

In a large serving bowl, combine the first four ingredients. Drizzle with dressing; toss to coat. Refrigerate leftovers. Serves 10

Just in Case Fruit Salad

a can of Del Monte fruit cocktail drained —save a little juice for after
a container of cool whip
a small bag of Jet Puffed mini marshmallows
bananas, sliced

mix all together -- if it looks a little dry add some fruit cocktail juice -- a little
bit at a time to your own liking (you don't want it watery!) you can add Baker's
Angel Flake coconut too if desired. Serves 8-10

Switchel

1 c boiling water
1 T honey
1 T herb vinegar (made with Heinz apple-cider vinegar)

Fill a cup with boiling water to dissolve the honey. Serve hot or iced for a
low-calorie, wine like drink. In days of yore, this energy refresher was drunk
as a thirst quencher. It also acts as a diuretic, and its potassium gives added
energy. Serves: 1

❧ SEPTEMBER ❧

**Overall Theme: Sunflowers, Apples,
(or whatever items your child returning to school likes)
Colors: Red, Black, White, Yellow**

BACK TO SCHOOL

Apple Peanut Crumble
(great after school snack)

4 or 5 cooking apples, peeled and sliced
2/3 cup Dominos brown sugar, packed
1/2 cup Bob's Red Mill all purpose flour
1/2 cup Quaker quick-cooking rolled oats
1/2 t cinnamon
1/2 t nutmeg
1/3 c butter, softened
2 T Smart Balance peanut butter

Place apple slices in slow cooker. In medium bowl, combine sugar, flour, oats, cinnamon, and nutmeg. Mix in butter and peanut butter with pastry blender or fork. Sprinkle over apples. Cover pot and cook on low for 5 - 6 hours. Serve warm; plain or with ice cream. Serves 4-5

Welcome Back To School Bag

Place all of the items in a brown paper bag with an apple stamped on the front.
Fold down the top and punch two holes then tie them with a ribbon.
Include this note: **This is your reminder bag.**

The **HERSHEY'S HUG** is to remind you that everyone
needs a hug from time to time even Mom and Dad
If you need one, please let the teacher know.
The **SMARTIE** is to remind you that everyone in your class
will be learning a lot and getting smarter every day.
The **NABISCO LIFE SAVER** is to remind you that you can go
to any adult in your school if you need someone to help you.
The **TISSUE** is to remind you to dry the tears of a friend if they need it.
The **ERASER** is to remind you that we all make mistakes and it is okay.
The **STARBURST** is to remind you that each
student in your classroom is a star.
The **SOCCER STICKER** is most important. It reminds us
to stick together and work as a team to reach our goal.

Hope this helps. ------------*Love, Mom & Dad*

Note: author unknown

Labor Day

Labor Day, the first Monday in September, is a creation of the labor movement and is dedicated to the social and economic achievements of American workers. It constitutes a yearly national tribute to the contributions workers have made to the strength, prosperity, and well-being of our country. More than 100 years after the first Labor Day observance on Tuesday September 5, 1882, in New York City, there is still some doubt as to who first proposed the holiday for workers.

In 1884, the first Monday in September was selected as the holiday, and the Central Labor Union urged similar organizations in other cities to follow the example of New York and celebrate a "workingmen's holiday" on that date.

Barbecued Ribs

7 1/2 to 9 lbs pork spareribs, cut into 2 - 3 rib pieces
3/4 c water, divided
Kraft Barbecue Sauce

Arrange one-third of ribs at a time in single layer in 12 x 8 inch baking dish or 3 qt casserole, overlapping slightly as needed. Add 1/4 c water; cover tightly with plastic wrap. Microwave at High 5 minutes. Reduce power to 50%. Microwave, covered, 15 to 20 minutes, turning ribs over once. Drain. Repeat twice with remaining ribs. Place on grill over hot charcoal. Cook until fork tender, basting with barbecue sauce. Serves: 10-12

Microwaved Corn on the Cob

Arrange **4 unhusked ears of corn** on oven floor with space between. No preparation is needed. Microwave 15 minutes turn over and rearrange every 4 minutes. Let stand 5 minutes. Husk corn after standing. Using paper napkin, hold corn with tip pointing down. Pull back leaves carefully to avoid steam. Grasp silk in other hand and pull sharply. Serves: 10-12

Baked Beans Made Easy

4 slices Black Label bacon
1/2 c chopped onion
2-16 oz cans Van Camps pork and beans
2 T Dominos packed brown sugar
2 T Heinz ketchup
1 T Lea & Perrins Worcestershire sauce
1 T French's prepared mustard

Place bacon in a 1 1/2 qt. casserole. Cover with paper toweling. Micro-cook till crisp, 3 1/2 to 4 min. Remove bacon, drain. Reserve about 3 T drippings in casserole. Crumble bacon and set aside.

Micro-cook chopped onion in reserved drippings till tender, 2 min. Stir in pork and beans, brown sugar, ketchup, Worcestershire sauce, and prepared mustard. Cook, uncovered, till bubbly, about 10 min. Stir twice. Top with bacon. Serves: 6

Coleslaw

Combine the following:

1/3 c Hellman's Mayonnaise
1 T Heinz vinegar
2 t Dominos sugar
1/2 t salt
1/2 t celery seed
3 c cabbage, shredded

Serves: 6-8

Frozen Cucumber Pickles

4 c cucumbers, sliced or diced
2 c onions
4 t salt
1 c Dominos sugar
1/2 c Heinz vinegar
1 t dill seed

Cut up cucumbers and onions in plastic bowl. Sprinkle with salt. Add cold water to cover. Let sit 2 hours, stirring 2 or 3 times. Drain off water. Do not rinse. Return to bowl and add sugar, vinegar and dill seed. Let set 30 or 40 minutes. Pack in jars. Seal tight and freeze. Makes 2 pints.

Apple Cake w/Honey Frosting

1 1/2 c Bob's Red Mill all-purpose flour
1 1/4 c packed Dominos brown sugar
1 1/2 t Calumet baking powder
1 1/2 t ground cinnamon
1 t Arm & Hammer baking soda
1/4 t ground nutmeg
1/4 t ground cloves
2 c peeled, finely shredded apple
3/4 c Crisco vegetable oil
4 eggs
1/4 c finely chopped Good Sense nuts

Place all ingredients in large bowl. Blend at low speed, scraping bowl constantly. Beat at medium speed 2 minutes, scraping bowl occasionally. Divide batter between two 8 x 8 in. baking dishes.

Place one dish at a time on inverted saucer in oven. Microwave at 50% 6 minutes. Increase power to High. Microwave 1 to 4 minutes. Or until top springs back when touched lightly. Let stand directly on counter 5 to 10 minutes. Cool and frost. Serves: 10-12

Honey Frosting

1/2 c packed Dominos brown sugar
1/2 c butter
1/2 c honey
4 c Dominos powdered sugar
2 t vanilla
1 to 2 T milk

In medium bowl combine brown sugar, butter and honey, Microwave at High 2 to 3 minutes, or until boiling, stirring after half the time. Boil 30 seconds longer. Stir in powdered sugar and vanilla. Add milk, 1 T at a time, beating until smooth and of spreading consistency. Cool before serving.

☙ OCTOBER ❧

Overall Theme: Leaves, Pumpkins, Gourds, Scarecrows
Colors: Fall colors

COLUMBUS DAY

Many countries in the world celebrate the anniversary of Christopher Columbus' arrival in America which occurred on October 12, 1492.

Columbus Day first became an official state holiday in Colorado in 1906, and became a federal holiday in 1934. Since 1971, the holiday has been fixed to the second Monday in October.

Celebrating Columbus Day

Consider incorporating a color theme of ocean blue and white. Set the table with ocean blue linens and white plates. A bowl of water with floating candles surrounded by seashells would make a nice centerpiece.

Poor Man's Lobster

2 (1-lb) blocks frozen haddock fillets, thawed enough to cut
   (about 1 hr at room temp)
2 c water
2 t salt
3 T Heinz apple cider vinegar
6 T lightly salted butter
1/2 t paprika
Lemon wedges or halves

Cut each block of fillets into 12 equal chunks, each about 1-1/4 inches square. In a medium-sized saucepan bring water, vinegar and salt to a boil over moderately high heat. Add fish chunks, reduce heat to moderate and simmer 15 - 20 minutes, until fish is opaque in center. Choose a broiler proof skillet or dish large enough to hold the fish in a single layer and melt the butter in it. Remove fish from liquid with a slotted spoon and add to butter; sprinkle fish with paprika and spoon butter over it. Broil 3 to 5 inches from heat source for about 4 minutes, spooning butter over fish once. Garnish with lemons. Serves 6

Serve with cooked brown rice, peas, and cooked apples sprinkled with Dominos brown sugar.

OKTOBERFEST

A time when the Germans celebrate their faith and freedom

Root Beer: To each guest, serve 1 1/2 c root beer, icy cold, in frosted mugs or beer steins. Serves 8

Hot Dutch Potato Salad

4 slices Black Label bacon
1/8 t pepper
1/2 c chopped onion
1 t Dominos sugar
1/2 c chopped bell pepper
1 egg
1/4 c Heinz vinegar
1 quart hot, cubed, cooked potatoes
3 hard boiled eggs
1/4 c grated raw carrot

Dice bacon and pan fry. Add chopped onion and pepper. Cook 3 minutes. Add vinegar, salt, pepper, sugar and beaten egg. Cook slightly. Add cubed potatoes, grated carrot and diced hard-cooked eggs. Blend and serve hot. Serves 8

Franks 'N' Dip

1/3 c Heinz ketchup
1/3 c Del Monte chili sauce
2 t Manischewitz prepared horseradish
2 t Smucker's low-calorie jelly, any flavor
6 oz Ball Park Frankfurters, cut into 24 equal pieces

In small saucepan combine ketchup, chili sauce, horseradish, and jelly. Add frankfurters; stir to coat. Cook over medium heat, stirring occasionally, until frankfurters and sauce are heated throughout. Transfer to chafing dish. Serve with toothpicks. Serves 8

Harvest Day - Barnyard Bash

Centerpiece: Flickering Luminaries

Invitations: Cut out animal shapes on construction paper and write the party information on these. Hand deliver to your guests.

Decorations: bales of hay, bunches of dried cornstalks, autumn leaves, pumpkins, gourds, and dried corncobs. Serve food in western bandanas attached to sticks. Be sure to make a scarecrow. Carved out pumpkins make great serving dishes or chip bowls.

Fall Harvest Games and Activities

Corn Husking Race: Give each child 4 ears of unhusked corn and race to see who can have all of their corn husked first.

Floating Pumpkins: Number the bottom of the small gourds that look like miniature pumpkins and float them in water for the children to choose one for small prizes.

Musical Bales: Play musical chairs with bales of straw instead of chairs. A scarecrow in the center makes a fun decoration.

Turkey In The Straw: Fill a wading pool with straw and hide a small picture of a turkey in it for groups to dig through to see who can find it first.

Pumpkin Race: Set up starting and finish lines and have the children race to see who can get their pumpkin over the finish line first using only their feet to slide the pumpkins along. No kicking the pumpkins like footballs.

The Classic Apple Dunking:
Need: Apples, Water, A deep pan or a half barrel, Lots of kids
You can blindfold the players or not. Put the water and apples in the barrel. Without using hands the players must pick up an apple with their teeth! (If you wear glasses then don't forget to take them off.)

Barnyard Bash Bites

Dinner in a Pumpkin

1 small to medium pumpkin
1 4-oz can sliced mushrooms, drained
1 onion, chopped
3/4 c Swanson's chicken broth
1 c Coffee Rich creamer
2 T Crisco vegetable oil
1 8-oz can sliced water chestnuts, drained
1 1/2 to 2 lbs ground beef
1 1/2 c Uncle Ben's cooked brown rice
2 T LaChoy soy sauce
2 T Domino's brown sugar

Cut off top of pumpkin; clean out seeds and pulp. Save seeds for toasting later. In a large skillet, sauté onion in oil until tender; add meat and brown. Drain drippings from skillet. Add soy sauce, brown sugar, mushrooms, broth and creamer; simmer 10 minutes, stirring occasionally. Add cooked rice and water chestnuts. Spoon mixture into pumpkin shell. Replace pumpkin top and place entire pumpkin, with filling, on a baking sheet. Bake for 1 hour in 350° F oven or until inside meat of pumpkin is tender. Put pumpkin on a plate; remove top and serve. For your vegetable, scoop out cooked pumpkin and serve. Serves 6.

Roasted Pumpkin Seeds

3 T of Crisco vegetable oil

Scoop out the insides of the pumpkin and rinse the seeds. Dry them and then fry them in a frying pan for 15 minutes. Make sure you stir them a little. Dry the oil with a towel. You can add salt if you wish.

Sloppy Joes

1 lb lean ground beef
1 c chopped onion
1/4 c chopped Vlasic dill pickle
1/2 c Heinz ketchup
1/4 c honey
1/4 c Contadina tomato paste
1/4 c French's prepared mustard
2 t Heinz apple cider vinegar
1 t Lea & Perrins Worcestershire sauce
8 Food for Life hamburger buns

Cook beef and onion in a large skillet over med.-high heat 'til beef is brown and onion is tender. Drain. Stir in remaining ingredients except buns. Cook, covered, 5 minutes, or until heated through. Spoon meat mixture onto bottoms of buns. Cover with tops of buns. Serves 8.

Crockpot Caramel Apples

In crockpot, combine **2- 14 oz pkg caramels** and 1/4 **c water**. Cover and cook on high for 1 to 1 1/2 hours, stirring frequently. Wash and dry **8 med. apples**. Insert stick into stem end of each apple. Turn control on low. Dip apple into hot caramel and turn to coat entire surface ----Holding apple above pot, scrape off excess accumulation of caramel from bottom apple. Place on greased wax paper to cool. Serves 8.

Peanut Butter Apple Dip

1 8 oz pkg Philadelphia cream cheese, softened
1 c Smart Balance peanut butter
1 c packed Dominos brown sugar
1/4 c milk
4 apples, cut into wedges

In a mixing bowl, combine the first four ingredients; mix well. Serve with apples. Store in the refrigerator. Makes 2-2/3 cups.

Haystacks

Melt **12 oz butterscotch bits** and add **1 c Planter's peanuts** to melted mixture. Stir in **1 can Chinese noodles**. Mix and drop with spoon onto waxed paper to harden. Serves 8.

Spice Bags for Warm Autumn Drinks

8 sticks cinnamon, broken into small pieces
2 whole nutmegs, crushed
1/3 cup minced dried orange peel (or 1/4 cup ground)
1/3 c whole cloves
1/4 cup whole allspice berries

Combine all the ingredients in a bowl, tie in sachets of 1T each in a double thickness of cheesecloth; transfer to an airtight container. One sachet of the mixture will flavor 1 quart of cider, tea or wine.

To use, simmer 1 quart of chosen beverage with 1 sachet for 20 minutes; ladle into mugs.

A jar of these packets with instructions for use also make a nice gift.

৪৩ NOVEMBER ৫৯

**Overall Theme: Corn Stalks, Hay Bales,
Pumpkins, Gourds, Scarecrows
Colors: Fall colors**

VETERANS DAY

*World War I known as "The Great War" officially ended when the Treaty of
Versailles was signed on June 28, 1919, in the Palace of Versailles outside the
town of Versailles, France. However, fighting ceased seven months earlier when a
temporary cessation of hostilities, between the Allied nations and Germany went
into effect on the eleventh hour of the eleventh day of the eleventh month. For
that reason, November 11, 1918, is generally regarded as the end of "the war to
end all wars."*

*In November 1919, President Wilson proclaimed November 11 as the first
commemoration of Armistice Day. The original concept for the celebration was
for a day observed with parades and public meetings and a brief suspension of
business beginning at 11:00 a.m.*

*Armistice Day was a day set aside to honor veterans of World War I, but in 1954,
after World War II had required the greatest mobilization of armed services in the
Nation's history; after American forces had fought in Korea, the 83rd Congress,
at the urging of the veterans service organizations, amended the Act of 1938 by
striking out the word "Armistice" and inserting in its place the word "Veterans."
With the approval of this legislation on June 1, 1954, November 11th became a
day to honor American veterans of all wars.*

*Veterans Day continues to be observed on November 11, to preserve the historical
significance of the date, and to help focus attention on the important purpose of
Veterans Day: A celebration to honor America's veterans for their patriotism, love
of country, and willingness to serve and sacrifice for the common good.*

Patriotic Blueberry and Strawberry Fluff

2 – 3 oz pkgs strawberry gelatin (plus ingredients as called for on package)
1 c Breakstone sour cream
12 oz Cool Whip, thawed
2 c chopped unsweetened strawberries
2 c blueberries

Prepare gelatin according to package directions. Refrigerate until set to gel state.

Remove from refrigerator and whip with mixer. Add sour cream and whipped topping. Fold in blueberries and strawberries. Lightly set again. Store dessert in refrigerator.

Optional: Top with additional Cool Whip, strawberries and blueberries.

White Grape Juice Punch w/Blue & Red Cubes

2 quarts white grape juice
1 quart ginger ale

Right before serving, pour together both ingredients (already chilled).

Add frozen fruit ice cubes. Some cubes frozen with strawberries and some with blueberries.

Getting ready for Thanksgiving Day

GETTING READY FOR THE BIG BIRD
PROJECT - HOW MUCH TURKEY?

Estimate 1 pound per person, which allows for seconds or leftovers. The larger turkeys are very chesty with lots of breast meat, so you will get more servings from a big bird.

If you need to cook more than 1 turkey here's a suggestion. In one oven, roast a large turkey to present on the table; it can be carved as everyone admires it. In a second oven, roast some turkey parts. The turkey parts will only take an hour or two to roast and can be covered loosely with aluminum foil and keep them in a warm place until ready to serve. OR cooked the night before and reheated.

<u>Two Weeks Before:</u>

1. Make a list of everything you will need to purchase, borrow or get together. This includes extra seats, linens, place settings, candles, flowers, as well as all the ingredients for each dish you plan to serve.

2. Consider asking guests to bring a specific dish. Family members who love to cook will be delighted to be asked.

TIP: ask them to bring the food in a serving dish - ovenproof if it needs to be heated.

3. If ordering food, ingredients or dishes, order well in advance.

4. Invite someone you know who will be alone for Thanksgiving, to share with you and your family.

5. Send a thank you to people who've made a difference in your life: Send a note thanking a teacher, or a congressman who voted for something you believe in, a celebrity who is promoting a good cause, local people who are making a difference, and to anyone you love for being the person they are. "Thanks for being You".

Two Days Before:

1. Purchase as many items as possible.

2. If you are going to use place cards to avoid igniting old family feuds, now is the time to prepare them and to decide on guest seating.

The Day Before:

1. Prepare any desserts or side dishes.

2. Take a few minutes to work out a timetable or game plan.
TIP: work backward from when you want to serve the meal.

3. Enlist your family to help tidy and clean the house.

4. Start setting the table with linens, candles etc. and
start collecting together all the china, cutlery and dishes.

The Big Day:

1. Badger, beg or bribe your family to help with last minute chores.

2. Every child seven and up knows how to be a TV reporter. Send him off with a video camera and a set of questions to ask family or friends and then play it back for the family during football halftime or after dinner.

3. Assign tasks to each child or adult. For example, answering the door, taking coats, serving snacks, and clearing dishes.

4. Have ***Thanksgiving Brunch*** while watching Macy's Thanksgiving Day Parade.

5. If the weather permits have Thanksgiving dinner in a park, at a lake or in the backyard

6. Set the table. If you decide to have a kid's table, consider using a paper tablecloth and provide crayons. Not only will this keep them occupied, but who wouldn't feel delightfully naughty drawing on the tablecloth?

7. It is a good thing to give thanks unto the Lord and to sing praises unto thy name, O most High:

I thank you God for most this amazing day; for the leaping greenly spirits of trees and a blue true dream of sky; and for everything which is infinite which is yet. ~E E Cummings ~

See Thanksgiving Blessings.

8. Each person names one thing they are thankful for using letters in Thanksgiving. It's one of those times when we feel good for saying out loud what's right in our lives.

9. Adults can tell how they celebrated Thanksgiving as a child.

10. Fill the sink with soapy water. As soon as each course is cleared, soak the cutlery and dishes.

11. Organize yourself so that you and your family can take a walk, hike after the meal. Make the excursion in the spirit of thankfulness.

12. Finally, relax, enjoy and be thankful to have your family and friends with you on this special day.

THANKSGIVING BLESSINGS

"The Lord is my strength and my shield; my heart trusts in Him, and I am helped. My heart leaps for joy and I will give thanks to Him in song." Psalm 28:7

"You turned my wailing into dancing; you removed my sackcloth and clothed me with joy, that my heart may sing to you and not be silent. O Lord my God, I will give you thanks forever." Psalm 30:11-12

To show forth Thy loving kindness in the morning, and Thy faithfulness every night. Psalm 93: 1, 2

"Come, let us sing for joy to the Lord; let us shout aloud to the rock of our salvation. Let us come before Him with thanksgiving and extol Him with music and song. For the Lord is the great God, the great King above all gods. In His hand are the depths of the earth, and the mountain peaks belong to Him. The sea is His, for He made it, and His hands formed the dry land. Come, let us bow down in worship, let us kneel before the Lord our Maker; for He is our God and we are people of His pasture, the flock under His care." Psalm 95:1-7

"I will give thanks to the Lord because of His righteousness and will sing praise to the name of the Lord Most High." Psalm 7:17

"Enter His gates with thanksgiving and His courts with praise; give thanks to Him and praise His name. For the Lord is good and His love endures forever; His faithfulness continues through all generations." Psalm 100:4-5

"The sting of death is sin, and the power of sin is the law. But thanks be to God! He gives us the victory through our Lord Jesus Christ." 1 Corinthians 15:56-57

"But thanks be to God, who always leads us in triumphal procession in Christ and through us spreads everywhere the fragrance of the knowledge of Him." 2 Corinthians 2:14

"Thanks be to God for His indescribable gift (grace)!" 2 Corinthians 9:15

"Be joyful always; pray continually; give thanks in all circumstances, for this is God's will for you in Christ Jesus." 1 Thessalonians 5:16-18

"How can we thank God enough for you in return for all the joy we have in the presence of God because of you?" 1 Thessalonians 3:9

Thanksgiving as a Holiday and
The First Thanksgiving

Thanksgiving is a holiday when families gather, give thanks, and celebrate the harvest with a special meal. As holidays go, it is quite calm and simple; a family day. It doesn't have the hype, gimmicks and materialism that surround some other celebrations.

Any American school child will tell you that the first Thanksgiving Day was the feast of the Pilgrims and the Indians. In December 1620, the Pilgrims landed in Plymouth, Massachusetts. They were ill prepared for the winter, with most of the ship's stores used up. Only 55 of the original 102 immigrants survived that first winter. The next spring, a Native American Indian called Squanto, who spoke English, befriended them. He introduced them to the local tribe, the Wampanoag, and their sachem (chief), Massasoit. This tribe welcomed the Pilgrims. Without the help of the Indians, they would never have made it through the following winter.

Squanto taught the Pilgrims about the corn, beans, and squash, which were the staples of the native diet. The newcomers learned that corn was to be planted when the bud of the white oak tree grew to the size of a mouse's ear. They were told to place three herrings in each corn hill to fertilize it, and to guard the plants from wolves and dogs that might dig up the fish. Squanto showed the Pilgrims where to fish and gather shellfish and how to make chowder. He told them which wild plants were useful for food and medicine. He showed them how to make corn meal and maple syrup.

Because of the Indian's assistance, the new settlers had a good harvest in the autumn of 1621, which would see them through the next winter. Governor Bradford proclaimed a day of thanksgiving and celebration of the harvest, and invited the neighboring 91 Indians to join in the feast.

The feast was more of a traditional English harvest festival than a true "thanksgiving" observance. It lasted three days. The gaming expedition might have brought home partridges, ducks, geese, and turkeys. We have no way of knowing whether turkey was part of the feast. The term "turkey" was used by the Pilgrims to mean any sort of wild fowl. We do know that the Indians brought venison. The rest of the dinner was very different than what we think of as traditional today.

Another modern staple at almost every Thanksgiving table is pumpkin pie. But it is unlikely that the first feast included that treat. The supply of flour had been long diminished. They had plenty of squash and pumpkins, which were probably just boiled. Corn could have been roasted in the fire, or ground into cornmeal and used to make "hasty pudding" or fried corn cakes. Plums, wild berries, including cranberries, would have been sweetened with honey or maple syrup to make a sauce for the meat. Nuts and dried berries were probably served as well. They might have enjoyed a salad of watercress and leeks. There was also no milk, cider, potatoes, or butter. There were no domestic cattle for dairy products, and the newly discovered potato was still considered by many Europeans to be poisonous. The meal would have definitely included some of the plentiful harvest from the sea: fish, lobsters, clams, and oysters. The Indians might have shared wine made from wild grapes.

Although the celebration of the Pilgrims and the Indians in the fall of 1621 is generally considered the first Thanksgiving, it was not an annual celebration until later.

It was Sarah Josepha Hale, a magazine editor, whose efforts eventually led to what we recognize as Thanksgiving. Finally, after a 40-year campaign of writing editorials and letters to governors and presidents, Hale's obsession became a reality when, in 1863, President Lincoln proclaimed the last Thursday in November as a national day of Thanksgiving. And in 1941, Congress finally sanctioned Thanksgiving as a legal holiday, as the fourth Thursday in November.

Today, Thanksgiving Day has lost some of its meaning. Most people buy all the fixings for their Thanksgiving dinner from the supermarket. Some city people are barely aware of the harvest or what it means. Some of the more spiritual aspects have also been eroded, and for some, Thanksgiving is nothing but a big meal wedged between football games.

THANKSGIVING FIXIN'S

BRUNCH

Pumpkin Bread

1 c Dominos sugar
1/4 c butter
1/4 c Mott's applesauce
2 eggs
1 c Libby's solid pack pumpkin
2 c Bob's Red Mill all-purpose flour
1/2 t salt
2 t Calumet baking powder
1/4 t Arm and Hammer baking soda
1 t ground cinnamon
1/2 c Sun Maid raisins
1 t grated orange rind
1/4 c Minute Maid orange juice
1/2 c Good Sense walnuts, chopped (optional)

Coat a 9x5x3-inch loaf pan with Crisco vegetable spray. Beat sugar, butter, and applesauce until creamy and light. Add eggs one at a time and continue to beat. Add pumpkin and mix until smooth. Combine flour, salt, baking powder, baking soda, and cinnamon. Stir into pumpkin mixture and mix until smooth. Add raisins, orange rind, orange juice and nuts. Stir well and pour into loaf pan. Bake at 350° F for 60-65 minutes. Makes 1 loaf, approx. 12 Slices

Pumpkin Butter

1 c cooked or Libby's canned pumpkin
1/2 c honey
1/4 c Grandma's molasses
1 T ReaLemon juice
3/4 t ground cinnamon

In a small saucepan, combine ingredients; mix well. Bring to a boil, stirring frequently. Reduce heat; simmer, uncovered, for 15 min. or until thickened. Refrigerate for at least 1 hour.

Cinnamon Dip

1-8 oz pkg Philadelphia cream cheese, softened
2 T milk
1 t vanilla extract
2 T Dominos brown sugar
1 t ground cinnamon
1/4 t ground nutmeg

Combine all ingredients and beat until smooth. Serve with fruit slices. Store in airtight container in refrigerator. Makes about 1 cup of dip.

Join Us This Thanksgiving for Dinner

Roast Turkey with Gravy

One 18-pound fresh Butterball turkey
About 12 cups of your favorite stuffing (see recipes that follow)
1 stick unsalted butter, at room temperature
Salt and freshly milled black pepper
2 1/2 quarts Homemade Turkey Stock (below),
Melted unsalted butter, if needed
3/4 cup Bob's Red Mill all-purpose flour

Position rack in the lowest position, and preheat oven to 325°F. Reserve the turkey neck and giblets to use in gravy or stock. Rinse the turkey inside and out with cold water. Pat the turkey skin dry. Turn the turkey on its breast. Loosely fill the neck cavity with stuffing. Using a thin wooden or metal skewer, pin the neck skin to the back. Fold the turkey's wings akimbo behind the back or tie to the body with kitchen string. Loosely fill the large body cavity with stuffing. Place any remaining stuffing in a lightly buttered casserole, cover, and refrigerate to bake as a side dish. Place the drumsticks in the hock lock or tie together with kitchen string.

Place the turkey, breast side up, on a rack in the roasting pan. Rub all over with the softened butter. Season with salt and pepper. Tightly cover the breast area with aluminum foil. Pour 2 cups of the turkey stock into the bottom of the pan. Roast the turkey, basting all over every 30 minutes with the juices on the bottom of the pan (lift up the foil to reach the breast area), until a meat thermometer inserted in the meaty part of the thigh (but not touching a bone) reads 180°F and the stuffing is at least 160°F, about 4 1/4 hours. Whenever the drippings evaporate, add stock to moisten them, about 1 1/2 cups at a time. Remove the foil during the last hour to allow the breast skin to brown.

Transfer the turkey to a large serving platter and let it stand for at least 20 minutes before carving. Increase the oven temperature to 350° F. Drizzle 1/2-cup turkey stock over the stuffing in the casserole, cover, and bake until heated through, about 30 minutes.

Meanwhile, pour the drippings from the roasting pan into a heatproof glass bowl or large measuring cup. Let stand for 5 minutes, then skim off and reserve the clear yellow fat that has risen to the top. Measure 3/4 cup fat, adding melted butter if needed. Add enough turkey stock to the skimmed drippings to make 8 cups total.

Place the roasting pan in two stove burners over low heat and add the turkey fat. Whisk in the flour, scraping up the browned bits on the bottom of the pan, and cook until lightly browned, about 2 minutes. Whisk in the turkey stock. Cook, whisking often, until the gravy has thickened and no trace of raw flour taste remains, about 5 minutes. Transfer the gravy to a warmed gravy boat. Carve the turkey and serve the gravy and the stuffing alongside. 18 Servings

Homemade Turkey Stock

Make Ahead: The stock can be prepared up to 3 days ahead, cooled, covered, and refrigerated for up to 3 days ahead or frozen in airtight containers for up to 3 months.

Turkey parts with lots of bone, like wings and backs, make the best stock. Use the turkey neck, heart, and gizzard in the stock, but not the liver (makes the stock bitter). When the stock is strained, you can retrieve the neck and giblets to use in gravy.

Browning the turkey parts first give the stock a rich color that will make a dark gravy. Cooking the vegetables brings out their flavor. The longer a stock simmers, the better, up to 12 hours. Make the stock in a 5 1/2-quart slow cooker. Transfer the browned turkey and vegetable mixture to the cooker, add the herbs, and pour in enough cold water to cover generously. Cook on Low, and the stock will barely simmer all night long, to make a clear, delicious stock. Makes about 2 1/2 quarts.

NOTE: If time is a factor, just simmer the stock for an hour or two--it will still be better than using water or canned broth to make your gravy. Or, make a pot well ahead of Thanksgiving and freeze it.

3 pounds Perdue turkey wings
Turkey neck and giblets (liver reserved)
2 T olive oil
1 medium each: onion, carrot, and celery rib with leaves, all chopped
6 parsley sprigs
1/2 t dried thyme
1/4 t black peppercorns
1 bay leaf

Using a heavy cleaver, chop the wings and neck into 2-inch pieces. (If necessary, ask the butcher to do this for you.) Using a sharp knife, trim away any membranes from the giblets.

In a large pot, heat the oil over medium-high heat. In batches, add the turkey wings, neck, and giblets and cook, turning occasionally, until browned on all sides, about 8 to 10 minutes. Transfer to a plate. Add the onion, carrot, and celery to the pot and cook, stirring often, until softened, about 6 minutes.

Return the turkey to the pot. Add enough cold water to cover the turkey by 2 inches. Bring to a boil, skimming off the foam that rises to the surface. Add the parsley, thyme, peppercorns, and bay leaf. Transfer to crockpot. Cook at a bare simmer for up to 12 hours. As needed, add more water to the pot to keep the bones covered.

Strain the stock through a colander into a large bowl. Let stand for 5 minutes, and then skim off the clear yellow fat that rises to the surface. If desired, remove the giblets, cool, finely chop, and refrigerate for use in gravy. The neck meat can be removed in strips, chopped, and reserved as well. Cool the stock completely before refrigerating or freezing.

COOK THAT TURKEY GOOD!

*** COOKING TIME ***

Weight (pounds)	Unstuffed/hrs	Stuffed/hrs
8 to 12	2 3/4 to 3	3 to 3 1/2
12 to 14	3 to 3 3/4	3 1/2 to 4
14 to 18	3 3/4 to 4 1/4	4 to 4 1/4
18 to 20	4 1/4 to 4 1/2	4 1/4 to 4 3/4
20 to 24	4 1/2 to 5	4 3/4 to 5 1/4

HOW TO CARVE A WHOLE TURKEY:

* **Let it Sit:** Once the bird is removed from the oven, it should stand for 20 to 35 minutes, depending on its size. This gives the juices a chance to soak into the flesh, allowing for succulent cuts of meat. Before you begin carving, have a warm serving platter ready and waiting for all the juicy white and dark meat you'll soon be slicing and digging into.

* **Remove the Legs:** Arrange the turkey, breast side up, on a cutting board. Steady the turkey with a carving fork. Using a sharp knife, slice through the meat between the breast and the leg. Next, using a large knife as an aid, press the thigh outward to find the hip joint. Slice down through the joint and remove the leg. Cut between the thigh bone and drumstick bone to divide the leg into one thigh piece and one drumstick.

To carve the drumstick, steady it with a carving fork and cut a thick slice of meat from one side, along the bone. Next, turn the drumstick over so that the cut side faces down. Cut off another thick slice of meat. Repeat turning the drumstick onto a flat side and cutting off meat, carving a total of four thick slices.

To slice the thigh, place it flat side down on a cutting board. Steady the thigh with a carving fork. With a knife, cut parallel to the bone and slice off the meat. Be sure to place all the cuts on warmed serving platter as you work.
* **Remove the Wings:** Before you carve the breast, the wings must be removed. Slice diagonally down through the edge of the breast toward the wing. Using a knife as an aid, press the wing out to find the shoulder joint; cut through the joint and remove the wing. Place the wing on the serving platter as is.

* **Carve the Breast:** To carve the breast meat, hold the back of the carving fork against the breastbone. Starting parallel to the breastbone, slice diagonally through the meat. Lift off each slice, holding it between the knife and fork, and place on the warm serving platter. Continue until you have carved all the meat on one side of the breast. Repeat, carving the other side of breast.

Herb Stuffing

1/2 c butter
1 med onion, chopped
2 stalks celery, chopped
4-6 cloves garlic, minced
2 t salt
1 t thyme
1 t rosemary
1 t sage
1 t black pepper
1/2 t savory
1 T dried parsley
1 c poultry seasoning
8 c stale Food for Life bread, broken into one-inch pieces

Melt butter in large skillet and add all ingredients except the bread and stock. Cook over medium heat until onions are soft. Pour into a large mixing bowl. Add bread and stock. Mix well.

To stuff a turkey: Fill main turkey cavity with stuffing.

To bake stuffing in pan: Preheat oven to 350° F. Butter a 15 x 10-inch baking dish. Transfer stuffing to prepared dish. Cover with buttered foil and bake until heated through, about 45 minutes. Uncover and bake until top is golden brown, about 15 minutes.

To cook in crockpot. Cook on high 1 hour and 4-6 hours on low.

Serves 6-8.

Cornbread Stuffing
1/2 t thyme
1/2 t sage
3/4 c celery, finely chopped
1/2 c onion, finely chopped
1/4 c parsley, chopped
4 c GF cornbread crumbs
1/4 c butter
1/2 t salt
1/2 t pepper

Cook celery, onion, and parsley in butter for about 4-5 minutes or until tender. Add thyme and sage. Mix lightly with other ingredients.

Cranberry Sauce
This recipe can be prepared up to 4 days ahead of time. Refrigerate until use.

3/4 c water
1/2 c Pillsbury Hungry Jack maple syrup
2 1/2 c fresh cranberries
1 T Minute Maid orange juice
1 t orange zest

Put the water and sugar in a saucepan and stir in sugar until dissolved, then add the cranberries and bring to the boil. Cook for 5-10 minutes or until the berries begin to pop. Chill until serving time. Makes about 4 cups.

Crock Pot Cranberries: Combine as above. Cover and cook on high 2 to 3 hours until some pop.

Corn with Roasted Garlic Butter

1 head garlic, halved across
1/4 c softened butter
6 t chopped parsley
1/2 t salt
4 ears freshly boiled corn, or frozen corn

Preheat oven to 400° F. Wrap garlic in foil; roast in oven for 40 minutes or until tender. Let cool; squeeze garlic pulp out of cloves into small bowl. Stir in butter, parsley and salt. Serve with ears of corn, or add to a bowl of cooked, drained frozen corn before serving.

Glazed Carrots

8 large carrots -- thinly sliced
1/4 c frozen Minute Maid apple juice concentrate, thawed
1 T grated orange zest
1 t Rumford cornstarch
1/8 t ground cloves

Steam carrots for 10-15 min or until tender. Combine apple juice, orange zest, cornstarch and cloves in a large saucepan and mix until smooth. Cook, stirring constantly until mixture has thickened and cleared. Add steamed carrots to the sauce, mix well and serve. Serves 8

Make-Ahead Frozen Angel Flake Biscuits

1 pkg Fleischmann's dry yeast
2 T warm water
1 c Crisco shortening
2 c Yoplait plain yogurt
5 c Bob's Red Mill all-purpose flour
4 T Dominos sugar
1 t Arm and Hammer baking soda
3 t Calumet baking powder
1 t salt

Cut shortening into dry ingredients. Add yeast and yogurt . Knead to dough consistency. Roll out to 1/2" thickness; cut with cutter. Melt butter. Dip biscuits in melted butter and fold in half. Freeze -- 12 to a pan. Do not thaw. Bake at 350° F 30 minutes or until brown.

Pumpkin pie
Make a homemade gluten-free pie crust using just three simple ingredients.

1/2 c Crisco shortening
1 1/2 c rice flour
4 T cold cold water

Cut shortening into rice flour until a crumb like texture forms. Add water. Work dough with hands until soft and form into ball.

Place dough in 8 inch pie pan and press it into the bottom and sides, use the back of a spoon or fingers. Set aside and prepare filling.

Filling:

1 c Dominos brown sugar
1/4 t cinnamon
1/4 t nutmeg
1 c cooked Libby's pumpkin
1 2/3 c evaporated milk
1/2 t salt
1/3 c water
2 T Bob's Red Mill all purpose flour
2 eggs, beaten

Mix together sugar, spices, salt, flour and stir into pumpkin. Add milk and eggs. Pour into 9-inch unbaked pie shell. Bake in 450° F. oven for 10 minutes. Reduce heat to 350° F. and bake 25 to 30 minutes, or until filling is firm.

A Menu for Two to Four People

Herbed Roasted Turkey Breast

1 bone-in Butterball turkey breast-about 3 pounds
2 slivered garlic cloves
1/2 t dried rosemary or a sprig of fresh
3 T honey
1 T French's Dijon mustard
1 T olive oil
1 T ReaLemon juice
1/2 t pepper
Salt to season

Make small slits in the top of the breast and insert garlic slivers and the fresh rosemary sprigs. If you are using dried rosemary, add it to the honey mixture instead. In a small bowl, combine honey, mustard, oil, lemon juice, dried rosemary (if using) and pepper. Brush herb mixture over the turkey breast. Sprinkle with salt. Place turkey in baking dish or roaster pan, meaty side up. Roast at 350° F for about 60 minutes. Baste every 10 to 15 minutes until done. Cooking time depends on the size of the breast, but a meat thermometer inserted into the thickest part of the breast should read at least 165 degrees. Allow to set while you finish the preparations - the carving will be much easier.

Herb Onion Stuffing

1 c finely chopped sweet onion, such as Vidalia
1 stick butter
5 c coarse fresh Food for Life bread crumbs
1 1/2 T chopped fresh tarragon
1 1/2 T chopped fresh chives
2 t salt
1 1/2 T chopped fresh flat-leaf parsley
1 t black pepper
3/4 c Swanson's chicken broth

Cook the onion in butter in a large heavy skillet over fairly low heat, stirring, until butter is melted and onion is slightly softened, about 5 minutes. Combine breadcrumbs, herbs, salt, and pepper in a large bowl and stir in butter mixture and gently stir in broth. If you like moister stuffing you may need to add more broth. Transfer stuffing to a buttered baking dish. Cover with foil and bake for 20 minutes with your turkey breast at 350° F, then uncover and bake until top is crisp and stuffing is heated through, about 20 minutes more.

Herb Buttered Zucchini and Carrots

Scrub **1 lb baby carrots** and **1 lb small zucchini**. Slice zucchini 1/8-inch thick and leave the carrots whole. To **½ cup boiling water** add **1 t salt, 1 t dried thyme** and carrots.

Cover and simmer about 10-15 minutes until carrots are still crisp-tender. Add the zucchini and mix well. Bring back to a boil and cover. Reduce heat and simmer about 5 minutes, until vegetables are tender. Drain and add 2 T butter, tossing gently to coat. This makes about 4 servings.

Pumpkin with Pecan Topping

2 eggs
2/3 c Dominos lightly packed brown sugar
1 t ground cinnamon
1/2 t salt
1/4 t ground nutmeg
3/4 c milk
1-14-oz can Libby's pumpkin puree (1 1/2 cups), not pie filling

Preheat oven to 325° F. Beat eggs in a large bowl. Stir in brown sugar, cinnamon, salt and nutmeg until evenly blended. Stir in pumpkin and milk until blended.

Pour pumpkin mixture into a glass pie pan and bake until the pumpkin filling seems set in the center when lightly jiggled, about 45 to 50 minutes more. Place on a cooling rack while making topping.

Topping:

1/2 c Dominos sugar
1/2 c Dominos brown sugar, lightly packed
1/3 c Karo corn syrup
1-1/2 c Good Sense pecan halves

In a large saucepan, combine sugars and corn syrup. Place over medium heat and cook, uncovered, stirring frequently, until sugar is completely dissolved, about 3 to 4 minutes. Remove from heat and stir in pecans. Evenly spoon over baked pumpkin mixture.. Place in center of preheated broiler rack. Watch carefully and only broil until the topping bubbles. It will happen quickly! Remove from oven and place on cooling rack. Can be served warm or at room temperature. Refrigerate leftovers for up to two days.

A Native American Feast

This meal can be prepared in the traditional way, by a fireside, using clean hot rocks and dropped into a clay pot, or in a Dutch oven. The main course can even be done in a large crock-pot, ensuring tender meat and very little work.

You can use any wild game meat; deer, elk, moose, caribou, or substitute a loin of pork or a piece of tender beef loin; whatever you have available.

Likewise, any mushroom will do, but wild mushrooms are preferred. (If using wild mushrooms, be absolutely sure you know what you are gathering and feeding to your family. Some are deadly.) Dried, rehydrated mushrooms are traditional and give a richer flavor.

In place of the wild onions and garlic, you could use domestic varieties, but you will be lacking flavor.

Venison and Wild Rice

3 lbs venison boneless loin
1 handful of wild onions
1/2 handful of wild garlic
2 qts. water
1 1/2 c dried mushrooms
2 t salt
1 1/2 c cleaned wild rice

Sear boneless loin, with fat trimmed, in just enough shortening to get the job done, allowing about 1/2 pound per person. If the loin is too long to place flat in roaster or Dutch oven, cut in two. (Sear all sides.) Add 1/2 cup cleaned, peeled wild onions (bulb end only), and 1/4 cup cleaned, peeled wild garlic. Sauté lightly. Add water, mushrooms, and salt. Simmer uncovered for three hours. Add wild rice, cover, and simmer for 20 minutes. Uncover and simmer for 20 minutes more or until rice is tender.

Baked squash with corn, wild greens, and hazelnuts

1 large sweet winter squash such as acorn
1 c fresh raw wild greens, such as lambs quarters
1/4 c wild hazelnuts
2 c sweet corn
1/4 c cranberries (optional)
1 T honey for each squash half
1T butter for each squash half

Slice the squash in half and remove seeds. Arrange on cookie sheet and bake 1/2 hour at 300° F. Meanwhile, chop the wild greens medium fine and chop the hazelnuts very fine. Add these to the corn. Add fresh cranberries for taste and color.

Spoon this corn mixture into each squash half. Add honey on top, then butter. Bake until the squash is tender and serve very warm.

Fry bread

4 c Bob's Red Mill all-purpose flour
1 T Calumet baking powder
1 t salt
1 1/2 c and a little more warm water
Crisco shortening to deep fry

Mix dry ingredients in a bowl. Add water and mix thoroughly. Knead, adding more water or flour as needed. Dough should end up elastic and soft but not sticky. Pinch off balls the size of a small peach. Pat back and forth in hands until about 1/2 inch thick. Melt shortening in heavy frying pan or heavy deep fryer. Heat until hot but not smoking. Carefully fry each bread in hot fat, turning till each side is golden brown. Drain on paper towels and serve hot with warm honey.

Wild blueberry cobbler

2 c dried wild blueberries (if using fresh or canned berries, use 4 c)
1/2 c honey

Topping:
1 1/2 c Bob's Red Mill all-purpose flour
1 t salt
1/4 c honey
2 T butter
1/2 c milk

Place blueberries in baking dish and sprinkle with honey. For the topping, mix all dry ingredients and honey then cut in butter and add as much milk as is needed to make a thick batter. Spoon this on top of the berries and bake for about 1 hour at 350° F.

Serve hot with Pillsbury Hungry Jack maple syrup, honey, or Cool Whip.

Consider the following Native American Wisdom:

"Every shining pine needle, every sandy shore, every mist in the dark woods, every clearing and humming insect is holy in the memory and experience of my people. Teach your children what we have taught our children, that the Earth is our mother. The rivers are our brothers, they quench our thirst and feed our children. The air is precious to the red man, for all things share the same breath--the beast, the tree, the man, they all share the same breath. And what is man without the beast? If all the beasts were gone, men would die from a great loneliness of spirit. This we know. The Earth does not belong to man; man belongs to the Earth. Man did not weave the web of life, he is merely a strand in it. Whatever he does to the web, he does also to himself. All things are connected like the blood, which unites one family. All things are connected."

-Sealth (Chief Seattle)

Vegetarian Thanksgiving

Vegetarian Gravy
Serve it over mashed potatoes or biscuits.

1 T butter
1/4 c minced onion
3 cloves minced garlic
4 T Bob's Red Mill all-purpose flour
4 c water or vegetable stock
2 t minced parsley
5 T low sodium LaChoy soy sauce
pepper to taste

Melt butter in a heavy skillet and sauté onion and garlic for about 2 minutes. Transfer to a bowl and wipe skillet clean. Add flour to skillet and cook, stirring constantly until flour gets brown and toasted. Add water or stock and soy sauce and cook, whisking constantly until mixture comes to a boil and thickens, about 5 minutes. Stir in onion/garlic mixture and parsley. Cook for one minute more. If gravy becomes too thick, thin with additional water or stock. Makes About 4 1/2 Cups.

Vegetarian Indian Corn Pudding

2 large eggs, beaten, or 1/2 c egg substitute
2 T finely chopped onion
2 T finely chopped red bell pepper
1/2 t salt
1/4 t ground mace
1/8 t ground white pepper
1 T butter
1-1/2 c skim milk
2 c fresh corn kernels or 1-15 oz can whole kernel corn, drained

Preheat oven to 325° F. Prepare a 1-1/2-quart casserole with nonstick pan spray. Combine the eggs, onion, bell pepper, salt, mace and white pepper in a medium bowl. Melt margarine in a large nonstick saucepan; stir in the milk and heat for 5 minutes. Add the egg mixture and corn; stir to mix well. Pour the mixture into the prepared casserole. Bake for 1 hour or until set. Makes 4 Servings

Vegetarian Cranberry Chutney

12 oz fresh cranberries
1 c peeled, diced apple
1 c Minute Maid orange juice
1/2 c chopped, dried apricots
1 t freshly grated ginger
1 t ground cinnamon
1/2 t ground cloves
4 T honey, or to taste

Place first 7 ingredients in a deep, heavy saucepan & bring to a simmer. Cook over low heat with lid slightly ajar for 20-25 minutes, or until liquid is mostly absorbed. Add honey to taste & simmer uncovered for another 5-10 minutes until thick. Cool to room temperature and store in sterilized jar, tightly covered but not sealed. Refrigerate. Bring to room temperature before serving. Makes 8 Servings

Candied Sweet Potatoes
For an extra kick add Jet Puffed marshmallows on top. Serve w/Cool Whip.

6 c of sweet potatoes, peeled and sliced
1/2 c unsalted butter, melted
1 c Dominos sugar
1/4 c of water

Arrange the sweet potato slices in a baking dish sprayed with nonstick spray. Combine the remaining ingredients in a bowl and spread evenly on top of the potatoes.

Sweet Potato Biscuits

1 3/4 c Bob's Red Mill all-purpose flour
2 t Calumet baking powder
1/2 t salt
3 T butter
1/3 c Musselman's apple juice
1 c well-mashed, cooked sweet potato
3 T honey
1/3 c finely chopped Good Sense walnuts

Preheat the oven to 425° F. In a mixing bowl, sift together the flours, baking powder & salt. Work the margarine in with a pastry blender or the tines of a fork until the mixture resembles a coarse meal. Add the apple juice, sweet potato, honey & nuts and work them in to form a soft dough. Turn the dough out onto a well-floured board and knead in just enough extra flour to make the dough lose its stickiness.

With floured hands, divide the dough into 16 equal parts. Shape into small balls and arrange on a lightly oiled cookie sheet, patting them down a bit to flatten. Bake for 12 to 15 minutes, or until a toothpick inserted into the center of one tests clean. Transfer the biscuits to a plate and serve hot.

Makes 16 Biscuits

Thanksgiving Ideas and Decorations

To make your Thanksgiving celebration special, begin with the table. A beautiful table is a sign of welcome and shows appreciation for each guest. Flowers, fruit, vegetables, pinecones, acorns and leaves are nature's gift to the Thanksgiving table. Low votive candles cast a warm glow. Paint names on miniature gourds or leaves with a gold marker and use as place cards. Use a hollowed pumpkin for a punch bowl or soup tureen. Use pumpkins, fall leaves, fresh fruit and candles for decorations.

Cornucopia Centerpiece

Cornucopia, pronounced kawr nuh KOH pee uh, is a horn of plenty, a symbol of nature's productivity. According to Greek mythology, it was one of the horns of Amalthaea, the goat who nursed the god Zeus when he was a baby. The horn produced ambrosia and nectar, the food and drink of the gods. In Roman mythology, the cornucopia was the horn of the river god, Achelous. The hero, Hercules broke off the horn in combat with Achelous, who was fighting in the form of a bull. Water nymphs filled the horn with flowers and fruit and offered it to Copia, the goddess of plenty. Stemming from these ancient mythologies, the cornucopia filled with fruits of the harvest became a symbol of gratefulness for the bountiful harvest and our Thanksgiving Day festivities.

1 cornucopia shaped basket or any basket you have on hand
Several branches of fall colored leaves
Raffia to tie a bow
About 12-1yd. strands Excelsior, straw or paper shreds in natural color
A variety of artificial or fresh fruits, mini-pumpkins, gourds and squash etc. to fill the basket

Arrange some of your leaf sprigs in a circle around a regular basket or in a fan at the opening of a cornucopia. Place the basket or cornucopia on the leaves and place the excelsior, etc. filler into the bottom of the basket to fill it at least 2/3 full, some pulled up around the edges. In the cornucopia shove it in and pull it out to form a base for your fruits and vegetables. Arrange the fruits and vegetables in a pleasing manner varying the colors and shapes that are next to each other. Clip some of the autumn leaves and tuck them in among the fruits and vegetables for accent and interest. Tie a bow in the center of your raffia streamers and attach it to the edge of the cornucopia or basket and if the basket has a handle on the handle.

Candy Corn Candle

Place a votive candle (in its glass cup) down inside a larger and empty clear cup and pour candy corn in the larger cup to surround the smaller votive cup.

Thanksgiving Potpourri

1 c sage leaves
1 c lovage leaves
1/2 c pumpkin seeds
1/2 c squash seeds
1 c Indian corn
2 c goldenrod
1/2 c sunflower seed
1 c evening primrose pods
2 c acorns
2 c hickory nuts
2 c basil leaves and flowers

This large quantity makes a colorful, crisp, and fresh-scented mixture that is decorative in open, glass containers for the holidays. After the festivities, it can be stored for later use as winter bird feed. The leaves will blow away, and the remaining nuts and seeds are attractive to foraging birds.

POPCORN

Popcorn was a surprise gift for the Pilgrims at the first Thanksgiving. According to legend, popcorn was discovered when a group of teenage American Indians threw some corncobs on the campfire.

Snap, Crackle
And Popcorn was born!
Make popcorn part of your
Thanksgiving tradition.

Nacho Popcorn

1 t paprika
1/2 t crushed red pepper
1/2 t ground cumin
1/4 c butter -- melted
10 c warm popped Jiffy Pop popcorn
1/3 c grated Borden's Parmesan cheese

In a small bowl, stir paprika, red pepper, and cumin into melted butter. Gently toss butter mixture with popcorn, coating evenly. Sprinkle with Parmesan cheese and toss till coated. Makes 10 cups.

Thanksgiving Traditions
*Who Gets The Wishbone?**

If you believe your wish will come true when you win the break in a wishbone contest, then you're following in the footsteps of civilizations dating back to the Etruscans, 322 BC and -- it started with a hen, not a turkey.

In those days, when a man wanted an egg he waited for the hen to announce the coming of her product. This made the animal mystical in that it could tell the future -- and that led to what became known as the "hen oracles".

If you lived back then, and wanted to receive an answer to an important question from these oracles, you would draw a circle on the ground and divide it into the twenty-four letters of the alphabet. Grains of corn were placed in each section, and the cock or hen was led into the circle and then set free. It was believed that the fowl would spell out words or symbols by picking up kernels of corn from the different sections.

For example, the first letter of a future husband's name would be the first kernel of corn picked. After writing the message, the fowl was sacrificed to a special deity and its collarbone was hung out to dry.

Then, you'd get to make a wish on the bone. Then two other people got a chance to make a wish by snapping the dried bone in the same way we do now, with each one pulling on an end. The person with the larger end of the bone got the wish -- and it became known as a "lucky break." The Romans brought the wishbone tradition with them when they conquered England, and that's how we got it.

ᔥ DECEMBER ᔥ

Overall Theme: Poinsettias and Holly
Colors: Red, Green, and Gold

Celebrating All December Long

Dec. 1 - Personalized Advent Calendar: Put your own messages behind the windows of store-bought Advent calendars. These messages might say, "I love you," give locations of secret hidden treats, or name a favor that the receiver may claim that day.

Dec. 2 - Christmas Dishes: Bring out any Christmas dishes and serving pieces. Use them every evening until the Christmas holidays are over.

Dec. 3 - Deck the Halls: Set aside one Saturday when the whole family helps put up all the house decorations (everything but the tree). Hang all the garlands, house lights, wreaths, and stockings and don't forget the mistletoe! Have carols on the stereo and chili in the crockpot. Then when all the decorating is completed, let your children invite some friends to join the family for dinner and a chance to admire the day's decorating work.

Dec. 4 - Christmas Greetings: Play Christmas music in the background on the telephone answering machine during the holidays.

Dec. 5 - St. Nick's Stocking: Hang St. Nick stockings early in the morning on the day before St. Nick's arrival (December 6). Throughout the day, each person in the family sneaks to the stockings and puts a gift in the other family member's stockings. These surprises to be discovered upon wakening on St. Nick's Day.

Dec. 6 - Cookie Exchange Party: Get together with a group of friends and bake cookies to exchange.

Cookie Exchange Party

Crockpot Hot Apple Cider

1 gallon Mussleman's apple cider or juice
12 whole cloves
3 sticks cinnamon
2 whole nutmegs
2 large pieces crystallized ginger

Place all ingredients in crockpot. Heat on high for 2 hours, and on low to keep warm until ready to serve. Makes about 20 servings. Keep another batch ready to go in the kitchen in a second crockpot or in a large pan on the stove simmering at the lowest temperature.

Snickerdoodles

Mix together until creamy:
1 c Crisco butter flavored shortening
2 eggs
1 1/2 c Dominos sugar

In another bowl, mix together:
2 3/4 c Bob's Red Mill all purpose flour
2 t cream of tartar
1 t Arm and Hammer baking soda
1/2 t salt

Next combine and mix all ingredients together. Chill dough for an hour.

Mix together: 1 t cinnamon and 1/4 c sugar

With the palms of your hands, roll cookie dough into small 1-inch balls. Roll each ball in sugar and cinnamon mix, covering completely. Place 2-inches apart on ungreased cookie sheet. Bake at 400° F for 8 to 10 minutes.

Chocolate Chip Cookies

8 oz unsalted butter, softened
1 t salt
2 t vanilla
3/4 c Dominos sugar
3/4 c firmly packed Dominos brown sugar
2 large eggs
1 ¼ c sorghum flour
1 c white rice flour
1 t Arm and Hammer baking soda
2 c Good Sense walnuts, broken (optional)
2 c Hershey's semi-sweet chocolate chips

Preheat oven to 375° F. Line baking sheets with parchment paper or grease pans lightly. Beat butter until soft and fluffy. Add salt, vanilla, and both sugars. Beat until smooth. Add eggs and beat.

Combine both flours and baking soda. Add half the flour mixture to the butter mixture and beat on low. Scrape down bowl with a rubber spatula. Add remaining flour. Fold in walnuts and chocolate chips. For best results, chill mixture for 2 hours.

Scoop into heaping tablespoon-size balls and set, 2 inches apart, on baking sheets. Flatten to about 1/2-inch thickness and bake 12-14 minutes or until browned all over. These cookies should be crisp; do not under bake. Let baked cookies stand a few minutes before transferring to a wire rack to cool completely. These freeze well. Makes 3 dozen cookies.

Peanut Butter Cookies

1 c Dominos light brown sugar
1 c Smart Balance peanut butter
1 egg

Mix together, roll out into small balls, and press balls with fork. Bake at 350° F for 9 to 12 minutes.

Peanut Butter No-Bakes

Cook these together in a large saucepan:

1 c Dominos sugar
1/2 c milk
2T Hershey's cocoa
1 t vanilla

Bring to boiling point and boil for 1 minute.

Then add:
1 1/2 c Quaker quick oats
2 T Smart Balance peanut butter

Stir these into cocoa mixture. Turn off heat right away. Stir for 1 minute. Now: Drop mixture by spoonfuls on wax paper. Work fast. These cookies set very quickly. Let cool and remove to plate or cookie jar. Serves: 8-10

Coconut Macaroons

1-14 oz pkg Baker's Angel Flake coconut
1 -15 oz can Eagle sweetened condensed milk
2 t vanilla or almond extract

Heat oven to 325° F. In medium bowl, mix the above ingredients. Drop dough by tablespoonful 2 inches apart onto a greased and floured cookie sheet. Bake for 13 to 17 minutes or until set and lightly browned. Immediately remove from cookie sheet. Makes 1 dozen cookies

Snowballs

1 stick butter
3 T Dominos powdered sugar
1 c Bob's Red Mill all-purpose flour, sifted
1 c finely chopped Good Sense walnuts

Cream butter and powdered sugar until fluffy. Stir in flour gradually, then walnuts until well blended. Chill several hours or until firm enough to handle.

Roll dough, 1 teaspoon at a time, into marble-size balls between palm of hands; place 2-inches apart onto ungreased cookie sheets. Bake 325° F for 20 min. or until lightly golden. Cool cookies on cookie sheets for 5 min; remove carefully and roll in powdered sugar. Store in container with tight fitting cover. Makes 4 dozen.

Sugar Cookies

3/4 c Crisco butter flavored solid shortening
1 c Dominos sugar
2 eggs
1 t vanilla
2-1/4 c Bob's Red Mill all-purpose flour
1-1/2 t Calumet baking powder
1/4 t salt

Cream shortening, sugar, eggs and vanilla in large mixer bowl at medium speed of electric mixer until light and creamy. Combine flour, baking powder and salt. Add to creamed mixture, mixing on low speed until well blended. Cover dough and chill 1 hour.

Preheat oven to 375° F. Roll half of dough at a time. Roll out dough on lightly floured surface to 1/4-inch thickness. Using a cookie cutter, cut in desired shapes. Place on ungreased baking sheets. Roll leftover pieces. Sprinkle with colored decorations or leave plain to decorate when cool. Bake for 8 - 10 minutes. Makes about 36 cookies.

Dec. 8 - Tree Decorating Party: Invite your friends to a great dinner party, and have each guest bring a tree ornament. After dinner, gather around and decorate the tree together. A wonderful variation would be to give the decorated tree to a needy family or a newlywed couple.

Dec. 9 - A Storybook Christmas: Each year, buy a new Christmas storybook for the family to read together for the remaining days until Christmas. Some favorites are "The Other Wise Man" and "A Cup of Christmas Tea". If your children are old enough, allow them to be a special part of this family time by designating certain nights for them to take turns as the reader.

Dec. 10 - Glad Tidings We Bring: Choose a night for writing letters to include with some of your Christmas cards. Have the whole family help by adding their own notes to each letter. Use attractive Christmas stationery for the notes, and embellish with stickers. Attach the following Christmas Aromatics to each card.

*Christmas Aromatics: Combine - **16 whole cloves, 3 pieces of cinnamon stick, 1 1/2 T pickling spice, and 1 t ground allspice.** Store in jar or plastic* bag. To activate add about 1 T to water in a potpourri simmering pot and heat gently. *Tie little bags of this with instructions on how to use it inside your Christmas cards.* Don't forget to make some for your own house!

Dec. 11 - Special Delivery: On the last Saturday before Christmas, play Christmas carols on the car stereo and hand deliver your Christmas cards to friends who live in your city. For that extra touch, include a small loaf of nut bread or a plate of homemade cookies.

Dec. 12 - Forget the Frenzy: Leave the Christmas frenzy behind today and take the family to a special Christmas movie or play. Top off the evening with an ice cream sundae at a favorite restaurant. Or just enjoy a quiet evening together around the fireplace -- add mugs of hot chocolate, pictures from past Christmases, and home movies for some old-fashioned fun.

Dec. 13 - The Gift of Time: Send a friend a postcard telling them about a special gift you plan to give them. For example: send a postcard saying "I'll pick up your child at 10:30 a.m. on December 15 for lunch and a movie so you can get some shopping done". Giving the gift of time to a busy mother can be the best gift of all.

Dec. 14 - A Note of Thanks: Place a pretty box of thank-you notes in each child's stocking to encourage your children to express their gratitude to relatives and friends.

Dec. 15 - A Christmas Puzzle: Start a new puzzle with a holiday theme on the first day of Christmas break from school. Make it a family project, but have guests to your home to contribute to it as well. Work toward the goal of completing your masterpiece by midnight on New Year's Eve.

Dec. 16 - Don't Open Until Christmas: A couple of days before Christmas, barricade the door to the room which contains the Christmas tree with large sheets of gift wrap. When the whole family has assembled to open gifts on Christmas morning or eve, the kids may run through the paper to see the brightly lit tree and all the gifts.

Dec. 17 - Festivities For Feathered Friends: Decorate a small potted tree branch with pine cones dipped in peanut butter and seeds and set this on the picnic table for the birds.

Dec. 18 - A Birthday Celebration: As Christmas Eve draws near, have the children bake a cake for baby Jesus. Let them do it by themselves, including the baking, frosting and decorating. The cake will be their own birthday gift to Jesus. This tradition reinforces to children the reason for Christmas and also gives mom time to put the finishing touches on her gift wrapping.

Author of the following invitation unknown.

You are cordially invited to
A BIRTHDAY CELEBRATION!!!

Guest of Honor: Jesus Christ

Date: Every day. Traditionally, December 25 but
He's always around, so the date is flexible....

Time: Whenever you're ready.
(Please don't be late, though, or you'll miss out on all the fun!)

Place: In your heart.... He'll meet you there. (You'll hear Him knock.)

Attire: Come as you are... grubbies are okay. He'll be washing
our clothes anyway. He said something about new white
robes and crowns for everyone who stays till the last.

Tickets: Admission is free. He's already paid for everyone... He
says you wouldn't have been able to afford it anyway... it cost Him
everything He had. But you do need to accept the ticket!!

Refreshments: New wine, bread, and a far-out drink He calls "Living
Water," followed by a supper that promises to be out of this world!

Gift Suggestions: Your life. He's one of those people who
already has everything else. (He's very generous in return
though. Just wait until you see what He has for you!)

Entertainment: Joy, Peace, Truth, Light, Life, Love, Real
Happiness, Communion with God, Forgiveness, Miracles,
Healing, Power, Eternity in Paradise, Contentment, and much
more! (All "G" rated, so bring your family and friends.)

R.S.V.P. Very Important! He must know ahead so
He can reserve a spot for you at the table.

Also, He's keeping a list of His friends for future
reference. He calls it the "Lamb's Book of Life."

Party being given by His Kids (that's us!!)! Hope to see you there! For
those of you whom I will see at the party, share this with someone today!

Dec. 19 - A Christmas Basket: On Christmas Eve, drop off a basket to an elderly couple, a single mother, or a financially-burdened family. Fill the basket with a coffee cake for Christmas breakfast, sliced cooked turkey for dinner, and a tablecloth and decorations to make the meals festive. Tuck a small wrapped gift amid the food for an extra surprise.

Dec. 20 - Fun and Games: Each year have your child give his or her grandparents a favorite board game for Christmas - one that your child does not have at home. Then the child and grandparents will have something fun to look forward to when the child comes to visit. To spark competition, put a chart in the game box to keep track of the winners.

Dec. 21 - Making Sweet Sensations: Make up a few batches of candy to give away to friends and family.

Fudge and Other Christmas Candies

Christmas Fudge

1-12 oz pkg Hershey's semi-sweet chocolate chips
1 stick butter
2 beaten eggs
4 c Dominos powdered sugar
1 t vanilla

Mix powdered sugar, eggs, and vanilla. Stir until smooth. Melt chocolate chips and butter over low heat, stirring constantly. Add sugar mixture to chocolate mixture and stir well. Pour into a buttered, 8-inch square glass pan. Score while soft. Refrigerate and cut when firm. Keep refrigerated or freeze.

Easy Fudge

1 can Eagles sweetened condensed milk
2 c Hershey's semi-sweet chocolate chips
1 t vanilla
Chopped Good Sense nuts (optional)

Put the milk and the chocolate chips together and microwave for 2 minutes. Stir a couple times. Continue to microwave (stirring every 30 seconds) until the mixture is smooth.

Remove from the microwave and add the vanilla and nuts. Pour into a buttered 8- inch square pan and chill. When hard, the fudge may be cut.

Peanut Butter Fudge

2 c milk
1 c Dominos sugar
1 c Smart Balance peanut butter (smooth or crunchy)
1-7 oz jar marshmallow crème
1 t vanilla

Stir sugar into milk over medium heat until sugar is dissolved, leave on medium heat without stirring until mixture reaches soft ball stage (it will start to turn a pale gold color). Remove from heat, immediately stir in peanut butter, marshmallow crème and vanilla, in that order. Stir rapidly because mixture will thicken quickly. When it is completely mixed and thickened, pour out into a buttered 8" square pan. Refrigerate for 30 minutes, and then cut into squares.

Candy Cane White Fudge

12 oz Hershey's white chocolate, coarsely chopped
14 oz can Eagle's sweetened condensed milk
1/4 c coarsely chopped CVS peppermint candies

Butter an 8-inch square baking pan; line bottom and sides with foil allowing foil to extend over sides of pan by about 1". Butter foil. Over medium-high heat in top of double-boiler or heatproof bowl set over pot of hot water combine white chocolate and condensed milk. Cook, stirring frequently, until melted and smooth, 5 minutes. Pour mixture into pan; sprinkle candy over top. Using knife lightly swirl candy into chocolate mixture. Refrigerate until firm, about 6 hours or overnight. Cut into 1" squares, diamond shapes or rectangles. Store in refrigerator. Makes 64 pieces.

Potato Candy

1 medium sized potato
Dominos powdered sugar
Smart Balance peanut butter (crunchy or smooth)

Boil a medium sized potato until done. Leave the skin on and peel it after it's cooked. Mash the cooked potato. Let it cool, then add powdered sugar until a dough forms. Roll the dough out to 1/4 inch. Spread peanut butter onto the rolled out dough. Roll the candy up and wrap it in wax paper or plastic wrap. Put it in the refrigerator to harden it up a little. Slice and eat.

Easy Microwave Peanut Brittle

1 c raw Good Sense peanuts
1 c Dominos sugar
1/2 c light Karo corn syrup
1 t vanilla
1 t butter
1 t Arm and Hammer baking soda

In a 1-1/2 quart casserole microwavable bowl, combine peanuts, sugar and light corn syrup, you do not need to stir. Microwave for 4 minutes on high. Remove and stir with a wooden spoon (it will seem dry). Microwave for another 4 minutes; remove and stir again. Add vanilla and butter, microwave for an additional minute. Remove and add baking soda-barely stirring into mixture. Pour onto greased baking sheet. Cool completely.

Dec. 22 - Grandparent's Ornament: As your family increases, give the grandparents a tree ornament with each new grandchild's picture on it. Or make them an ornament each year that includes a recent family photo. Involve your kids in creating the ornament -- they'll have fun making it, and the grandparents will treasure the gift all the more.

Dec. 23 - The Christmas Story: Gather your children before bedtime and read them the story of Jesus' birth, found in Luke, Chapter Two. Or for an illustrated Christmas story, read from a children's Bible or another book available from the library. On this special evening, make sure the children fall asleep knowing the reason we celebrate this season.

Dec. 24 - A Candlelight Service: Since it is often difficult for parents with young children to go to a candlelight church service on Christmas Eve, why not hold your own candlelight service at home? Give each family member a Scripture verse to read, then light some candles and sing your favorite Christmas hymns. After dad closes the service with a Christmas blessing, tuck the children into bed with pleasant thoughts of tomorrow.

Christmas Eve Dinner

Roast Tenderloin of Beef

6 lbs Hormel beef tenderloin
4 T Crisco oil
4 T coarse sea salt
4 T coarse ground black pepper
2 T coarse ground green pepper
2 T rosemary, crushed

On rack in roasting pan, bring roast to room temperature - 2 or 3 hours. Tie roast at 2-inch intervals to equalize thickness. On plastic wrap, coat roast with oil. Roll in seasonings. Let sit one hour. Preheat oven to 425° F. Roast tenderloin to internal temperature of 125° F, approx. one hour. Remove from oven and place on serving platter. Loosely tent with foil and rest at least 25 minutes. Carve about one inch thick and serve.

Cranberry Pork Roast

3 to 4 lb Hormel pork roast
1 c ground or finely chopped cranberries
1/4 c honey
1 t grated orange peel
1/8 t ground cloves
1/8 t ground nutmeg
salt and pepper

Sprinkle the roast with salt and pepper. Place in crock-pot. Combine the remaining ingredients; pour over the roast. Cover and cook on low for 8 to 10 hours. Makes 6 to 8 servings.

Cranberry Salsa

A delicious twist on cranberry sauce, a wonderful accompaniment to any grilled or roasted meat.

1-12 oz pkg fresh cranberries
1 large onion, chopped
2 Golden Delicious apples, peeled, cored, and chopped
1 c Dominos sugar
1 c golden Sun Maid raisins
1/2 cup plus 2 T water
3 T ReaLime juice
1 large garlic clove, minced
1/2 t ground cumin
1/2 t salt
1/2 red bell pepper, seeded and coarsely chopped

In a 3 to 4-quart pot, combine cranberries, apples, onion, sugar, and raisins, 2 T of the water, lime juice, garlic, cumin, and salt. Cook over medium-high heat until sugar dissolves and liquid begins to boil, stirring constantly.

Reduce heat to medium and simmer 7 minutes. Add bell pepper and simmer 3 minutes or until pepper is crisp-tender and mixture thickens. Remove from heat, stir in remaining 1/2 cup water. Store in the refrigerator up to one month. Makes about 4 3/4 cups.

Christmas Cauliflower

1 large head cauliflower (florets)
1/4 c diced red pepper
1-7.3 oz jar sliced mushrooms, drained
1/4 c butter
1/3 c Bob's Red Mill all-purpose flour
2 c milk
1 c (4 oz) shredded Kraft Swiss cheese
Paprika, optional

In a large saucepan, cook cauliflower in a small amount of water for 6 min. or until crisp-tender; drain well. In a medium saucepan, sauté pepper and mushrooms in butter for 2 min., stirring constantly. Remove from the heat; stir in cheese until melted. Place half of the cauliflower in a greased 2-qt. baking dish; top with half of the sauce. Repeat layers. Bake, uncovered, at 325° F for 25 min. or until bubbly. Sprinkle with paprika if desired. Serves: 8-10

Holiday Jell-O

2 pkgs of the small boxes of green lime Jell-O
1 jar maraschino cherries
8 oz pkg Philadelphia cream cheese

Prepare Jell-O as instructed on box and pour into container. Throw in cherries. Put in chunks of cream cheese, no bigger than one inch cubed. Place in refrigerator and serve when molded. Makes 10 servings

Ambrosia

1-20 oz can Dole pineapple chunks in juice
1 firm, large banana (sliced)
1-11 oz can Del Monte mandarin orange segments in syrup
1-1/2 c seedless grapes
1 c miniature Jet Puffed marshmallows
1 c Baker's Angel Flake coconut
1/2 c chopped Good Sense pecans
1 c Breakstone regular sour cream
1 T Domino's brown sugar

Drain pineapple and orange segments. In a large bowl, combine pineapple, mandarin oranges, banana, grapes, marshmallows, coconut and nuts. In small bowl, combine sour cream and brown sugar. Stir into fruit mixture. Refrigerate, covered at least 1 hour or overnight. Makes 6 servings.

Christmas Punch

2 qt Musselman's apple cider
2 c Dominos sugar
2 t whole allspice
2 t whole cloves
6 cinnamon sticks
1 qt Musselman's cranberry juice
1 pt Minute Maid orange juice
1 1/2 c ReaLemon juice

Combine cider and sugar in a large saucepan. Tie allspice, cloves and cinnamon sticks together in a porous cloth; add cider. Cover and simmer 15 minutes. Remove spices. Add remaining ingredients; simmer 10 minutes. Garnish with orange and lemon slices. Serve hot! Makes 1 gallon.

Coffee Punch

12 c extra-strong black Folger's coffee
1 1/2 c Domino's sugar
1- 5 1/2 oz can Hershey's chocolate syrup
2 T vanilla
3 quarts cold milk
3 quarts vanilla Turkey Hill ice cream

Brew coffee; transfer to glass container or bowl; add sugar, chocolate syrup, and vanilla. Place in refrigerator overnight. When ready to serve add cold milk and vanilla ice cream. Serves 40-50.

Dec. 25 - Prolonging the Joy: Instead of frantically opening all the gifts at one setting, why not spread the presents out over several days? How about opening only the gifts from friends on Christmas Day? Then over the next week, open the presents from family members, one each day, until the presents are gone. This allows children (and adults) to enjoy each present more fully, avoiding the mad rush for gifts on Christmas.

A HOLIDAY BRUNCH!

Scrambled Eggs and Cheese

12 eggs
4 T butter
1/2 t salt
Pepper to season
6 T half and half
Fresh chives
1 c finely grated mild Kraft Cheddar cheese

In a bowl, slightly beat eggs. Add the salt, pepper and cream, whisk briskly to mix. Heat butter in large skillet over low heat. Add the egg mixture and cook slowly. As the eggs just start to set, lift and stir. Continue to do this, adding the cheese as they begin to firm up. Remove from pan when they are no longer wet, but not browned. Transfer to platter and garnish with fresh snipped chives. This should be the last dish you prepare before serving guests.

Fresh Fruit Salad with Honey Cream Dressing

4 crisp apples, sliced, unpeeled
2 cantaloupes, cut up into chunks
2 kiwi, peeled and sliced
2 c seedless green and red grapes
2-16 oz cans Dole pineapple chunks, drained

Honey-Cream Dressing

1/2 c Breakstone's regular sour cream
2 c Breakstone's regular cottage cheese, creamed
2 c Yoplait plain yogurt
4 T honey
4 t ReaLime juice
2 t vanilla

Combine sour cream, cottage cheese, and yogurt. Mix will. Blend in honey and lime juice. To assemble salad: combine all fruit, except kiwi, in a large bowl. Garnish the top with slices of kiwi. Serve the dressing on the side with a small ladle so guests can add their own.

Breakfast Wassail

1-12-oz undiluted Dole pineapple juice concentrate
1-64-oz Musselman's cranberry juice
1-12-oz undiluted frozen Minute Maid lemonade concentrate
1-32-oz Musselman's apple juice
3 to 4 cinnamon sticks
1 qt. water, optional

Combine all ingredients in a large saucepan. Bring to a boil. Reduce heat; simmer 1 hour. Add water if desired. Serve hot or cold. Makes 4 quarts.

A Simple Holiday Buffet

The following recipes are for 12 because it is an average number of guests, but you can multiply the amounts as far as you need to. Let's start out with the tips, and then the recipes. The menu is simple, inexpensive and tasty.

Holiday Decorations are so simple for buffets. Use one large tablecloth over the buffet table and place sprigs of pine with red ribbon bows attached, and pinecones in small bowls along with potpourri, in-between the platters and bowls. Candlesticks are also very nice. You can also put phone books under the tablecloth to set some bowls higher than others.

Vegetable Christmas Tree Centerpiece

1 Styrofoam cone
Large round platter or plate
Lettuce, parsley or other greens to cover the cone & platter
2 small serving spoons
2 styles bottled Wishbone dressing
1 each large green and red Bell pepper with flat bottoms
Variety of vegetables, pickles, and cheese cubes, whole or cut in uniform sized pieces
Toothpicks
Small amount of floral clay
Plastic wrap and zipper bags

Cut a slice off the top of each pepper and remove the centers, wash, dry, cover with plastic wrap and place in refrigerator until serving time. Place a small amount of floral clay on the bottom of the Styrofoam cone and anchor it to the center of the platter. Using the toothpicks, pin the greens to the cone to completely cover and add more around the base to cover the platter. Cover with plastic wrap and refrigerate. Clean and prepare the vegetables etc. They should be left whole if small or cut so all pieces are about the same size.

Place a toothpick in each piece and place them in plastic wrap or zipper bags by kind and refrigerate. A few hours before the party arrange some of the veggies in spirals around the cone alternating colors by sticking the end of the toothpick into the cone. Arrange the red and green peppers one on either side of the cone on the bed of greens and fill with the dressings, a Ranch or Buttermilk style will look good in the red while

Raspberry Vinaigrette or Thousand Island will show well in the green. Place some of the remaining veggies on the platter with the toothpicks up. The rest can remain refrigerated to replenish as needed. This makes a pretty centerpiece for a buffet table.

Planning Tips

*Always have regular and decaf coffee hot and ready to serve. DO NOT run out. Angry mobs have been known to gather waiting for coffee.

*If people ask to bring food then LET them! In the case of our buffet menu, we have a wonderful fruit salad for dessert. If your guests ask, then request they bring holiday cookies or breads. Have clean platters and plates ready and waiting. Serve them near the fruit salad. Set up a smaller table as a dessert buffet for a nice touch

*If you have the budget to use nice disposable plates, napkins and tableware then do so. Otherwise, mix and match your own, and borrow some if you have too.

*Relax, and keep the mood light. There is no sense entertaining if you become overwhelmed and don't enjoy yourself. Ask your guests to bring their favorite Christmas music, and games. Be sure to have coloring books and kid's games on hand also.

The Buffet Menu:

Shaved Hormel Ham
Food for Life or Ener-G Rolls
Relish Tray
Vegetables and Dip
Fruit Salad
Oscar Mayer BBQ Cocktail Franks

Shaved Ham: Watch for sales on a nice, boneless ham. You will only need a half of ham, but a whole ham is less expensive per pound and will come in handy for lunches and other family meals. Ask at the meat counter to have it shaved, not sliced. Layer the ham on a nice platter; this will be your biggest dish. Garnish with green onions. Prepare ahead and wrap tightly with plastic wrap.

Rolls: I recommend already prepared bakery rolls that are assorted to save you time. Have at least a total of 2 dozen. You can serve these in napkin lined wicker baskets.

Relish Tray: A nice tray will have dill and sweet pickles, olives, some type of peppers, and green onions. However, IF you are really on a budget there is NOTHING wrong with both types of pickles and the green onions. These are inexpensive and often on sale. A divided dish works well for these.

Vegetables and Dip: This is a list of the vegetables you will need for approximately one dozen people, and a dip recipe follows. You may either use a platter set up for dips, or a large platter with a pretty bowl placed in the middle for the dip. Be sure to arrange the vegetables nicely, and mix the colors.

1 lb baby carrots or carrot sticks
1 lb bag a radishes
2 green peppers
2 cucumbers
small head of cauliflower

Cream Cheese Italian Dip

2 - 8 oz Philadelphia block cream cheese
2 envelopes dried Italian dressing mix
2 c Breakstone regular sour cream
2 T milk

Beat all items in a small mixing bowl with electric mixer until blended. Refrigerate. This makes 4 cups which may be too much, but it also makes a great chip dip. It's better to have too much than not enough!

Fruit Salad

Fruit:
2 large cans Del Monte fruit cocktail
1 medium can Del Monte mandarin oranges
1 can pitted dark red cherries (not pie filling)
1 large can Dole pineapple tidbits
1/4 c Baker's Angel Flake coconut
1/4 c chopped Good Sense walnuts

Dressing:
1 8 oz Philadelphia block cream cheese
1 small jar marshmallow cream
1 T Minute Maid orange juice
1/4 t nutmeg

Drain all fruit, and rinse cherries. Combine all fruit in a large bowl. Mix JUST the dressing ingredients together well with a whisk. Add to the fruit and gently mix with a wooden spoon.

NOTE: Bananas do NOT work well in this. You may substitute other fresh fruit.

BBQ Cocktail Franks

Large package Oscar Mayer cocktail franks (3 1/3 pounds)
1/2 small onion
Kraft BBQ sauce to cover, approximately 1 quart
1/2 green pepper

Chop the onion and green pepper into small pieces. Add to a crockpot with the franks. Cover with BBQ Sauce and mix together. Set the crockpot on low. These are the best when simmered for long periods of time, so start them in the morning if possible. Stir occasionally. Serve these directly out of your crockpot or transfer to a serving bowl just before eating.

Beverages: Know the people you are inviting. I would always have the hot coffee on hand to start and then add from there. Punch is always fun for adults and children. You can also serve hot chocolate heated in a crock pot. Use your imagination!

Wassail

Use very big pot:
8 c Red Rose tea (strong)
46 oz Dole pineapple juice
1 gallon Musselman's apple juice
1 large can Minute Maid orange juice concentrate
1 large can Minute Maid lemonade concentrate
1 c Dominos sugar
5 sticks cinnamon

In cheesecloth bag tie:
1 T whole cloves
1 T whole allspice
½ t ground cinnamon
¼ t ground cloves
water to taste (at least 2 cups)

Let simmer 1 hour or longer on stove on low heat. Float orange and lemon slices on top of wassail while simmering. Remove bag and cinnamon sticks before storing. Can be refrigerated for one week.

Dec. 26 - The Christmas Photo: Have a picture taken of your family by the decorated Christmas tree each year and display these pictures in a special photo album. Try to change one small thing on the tree each year, and then as you look back through pictures, see if you can find each of the changes.

Dec. 27 - Theme Card Collection: Save the Christmas cards you receive that pertain to a chosen theme, such as cards with angels, village scenes, antique toys, or Christmas trees. Opening cards each Christmas will be more exciting if you have a collection in mind. Set the cards from this collection in an area during the holidays for friends and family to enjoy.

Dec. 28 - Curing Christmas Blues: When all the relatives have left the grandparent's house after Christmas, the blues can act it. To brighten their days after your departure, encourage each guest to hide small "I love you" and "thank you" notes around the home for them to find in the days and weeks to come. These little discoveries will surely give Grandma and Grandpa a deserved lift in spirits.

Dec. 29 – Have an After Christmas Party. This is great for family and friends you don't see on Christmas Day.

Oyster Stew

NOTE: "liquor" in the context of this recipe does not mean alcohol, but rather the briny liquid in the oyster shell.

36 shucked oysters and liquor
1 qt light cream
8 T butter
salt
Lea & Perrins Worcestershire sauce
paprika

Remove the oysters from the shells; strain and reserve 1-cup of the liquor. Heat the liquor and cream in a saucepan. Melt the butter in another saucepan. When it froths, add the oysters and stir gently until they are hot and the edge begin to curl. Stir in the cream mixture, season to taste with remaining ingredients, and serve immediately. Serves 4

After Christmas Chicken

Combine **1-4 oz French's gourmet mustard** and **1 mustard jar of water**, paint **1 cut-up fryer chicken**. Arrange in a 9x13-inch baking dish. Sprinkle with **1-8 oz crushed pkg Energ-G herb stuffing mix**. Bake 350° F, uncovered, 1 hour or until juices run clear.

Holiday Ham Spirals

1-8 oz Philadelphia's block cream cheese
1/2 c finely chopped Sunsweet dried cherries
6 T crushed Good Sense pecans
5 T Hellman's mayonnaise
1 t spicy brown French's mustard
8 slices thin slices of Hormel ham

In a small bowl combine the cream cheese, cherries, pecans, mayonnaise and mustard; mix well. Spread mixture on ham slices and roll up jellyroll style; fasten with toothpicks. Allow to chill several hours. Remove the toothpicks and carefully slice into 1/4-inch pieces. Can be served on crackers or alone. Place on holiday platters for serving. Makes about 80 rolls.

Leftover Casserole

2-3 c turkey, chicken, ham or beef, whatever you have leftover
1-2 c gravy
2 c mashed potatoes
1-12-oz bag of mixed vegetables (or any kind you prefer),
    OR use leftover veggies
Leftover stuffing, if you have it, or use your favorite stuffing recipe,
    enough to top the casserole

Heat oven to 350° F. In a 9x13 pan spread the mashed potatoes in the bottom of the pan, layer meat and vegetables over the potatoes. Spread gravy over the top, and then top with leftover stuffing. If you don't have stuffing leftover, or don't care for it, you can put the mashed potatoes on top of the casserole to make a crust. Bake for approximately 30 minutes or until hot. Serves 4-8.

Vegetables and Pesto Dip

3 c fresh parsley, minced
1 1/4 c Kraft Parmesan cheese
1/2 c chopped Good Sense walnuts
1/2 c olive oil
2 cloves garlic
2 c Hellman's mayonnaise
2 c Breakstone regular sour cream
2 t seasoned salt
1/2 t black pepper

Vegetables:
2 lbs baby carrots
2 bunches red radish
2 cucumbers
1 bunch green onions
2 red peppers
1 bunch celery

Dip: Place first four ingredients in a blender. Process until mixture resembles coarse meal. Add remaining items and process until smooth. Makes about 6 cups

Vegetables: Clean, peel and slice the vegetables as necessary. Baby carrots can be left whole. Green onion can be trimmed with some green left on. The other vegetables can be cut into fairly good-sized pieces. Arrange in an attractive manner on a large platter with the dip in the middle. Garnish with parsley sprigs.

Karen E. Ruckman

Colorful Vegetable Salad

6 c broccoli florets
6 c cauliflowerets
2 c cherry tomatoes, halved
1 large red onion, sliced

Ranch Dressing Mix
1 T dried parsley, crushed
1 t dried dill weed
1 t onion powder
1 t dried minced onion
1 t salt
1/2 t garlic powder
1/4 t ground pepper

2/3 c olive oil
1/4 c Heinz vinegar

In a large bowl, toss the broccoli, cauliflower, tomatoes, and onion. In a jar with a tight-fitting lid, combine dressing mix, oil and vinegar; shake well. Pour over salad and toss. Refrigerate for at least 3 hours. Makes 20 servings.

NOTE: If you have leftovers to store, remove the onions as they become very soggy. The rest will store for several days.

Ambrosia Waldorf Salad

2 c fresh cranberry halves
1/2 c Dominos sugar
3 c miniature Jet Puffed marshmallows
2 c diced unpeeled apples
3/4 c chopped Good Sense pecans
1-20 oz can Dole pineapple tidbits, drained
1 c Cool Whip
Baker's Angel Flake coconut

Combine cranberries and sugar. In a large bowl, combine the marshmallows, apples, grapes, pecans and pineapple. Add cranberries and mix well. Fold in Cool Whip. Cover and chill. Sprinkle with coconut before serving.

Serves: 12-14

Steaming Hot Holiday Punch

3 c Musselman's apple juice
3 c Minute Maid orange juice
6 c Musselman's cranberry juice
3/4 c Pillsbury Hungry Jack maple syrup
2 t Dominos powdered sugar
1 1/2 t ground cinnamon
3/4 t ground cloves
3/4 t ground nutmeg
cinnamon sticks for garnish

Combine all ingredients in a very large heavy pan. Bring to boil, reduce heat and simmer for 10 minutes. Serve in mugs with cinnamon stick stirrers.

Dec. 30 - The New Year's Eve Photo: Gather the family for a picture at the end of every year. Have each person wear clothes significant to an important event in the past year -- a T-ball outfit for the first year on the team or a brownie scout outfit for the first year in scouting. Hold objects that pertain to the year's achievements or have the family stand around a new car for the picture. Frame this picture to hang on a special family history wall.

Dec. 31 - Epiphany Cookies: Bake and decorate star-shaped cookies to eat and give to friends on Epiphany (January 6). Put them in decorative bags with a note that says, "Wise men still seek Him".

In Italy, January 6th is a day long-awaited by many children. Children receive presents traditionally brought by the "Befana," a good old witch who comes into their homes through the chimney. This is the last day to the Christmas holiday in Italy.

Gift Giving Ideas

Sugar-Glazed Walnuts

1/2 c butter
1 c Dominos brown sugar
1 t cinnamon
1 lb Good Sense walnut halves (about 4 c)

Place butter in 1-qt casserole; microwave on high 1 minute or until melted. Stir in brown sugar and cinnamon; microwave on high 2 minutes (melt well). Add nuts and mix to coat; microwave on high 3-5 minutes. Mix well, and then spread onto waxed paper to cool.

Honey Pecan Mix

6 c Chex cereal
1 c mini Glutino pretzels
1 c Good Sense pecans
1/3 c butter
3/4 c firmly packed Dominos brown sugar
1/4 c honey
1 t vanilla

Coat a 9x13 baking pan with butter; add cereal, pretzels and pecans. Set aside. In a large saucepan, over medium heat, combine butter, sugar and honey. Bring mixture to a boil, and continue to boil 5 minutes, do not stir. Remove from heat and stir in vanilla. Pour syrup over cereal mixture, stirring until well coated. Baked at 250° F about 1 hour, stirring every 15 minutes. Let cool.. Store in airtight container.

Spicy Nuts

1 1/2 c whole Blue Diamond almonds
1 c each Good Sense pecan and walnut halves
2 T Crisco vegetable oil
2 t curry powder
2 t cumin
1/2 t cayenne pepper
1/4 t white pepper

Preheat the oven to 350° F. In a large bowl mix together the nuts and toss with the oil to coat evenly. Add the spices and toss to distribute evenly. Spread the nuts in a single layer on a baking sheet. Bake for 10 minutes. Salt to taste.

Last Minute Gift Ideas:
Computer to the Rescue!

Recipe Cards

Print favorite recipes on 4-by-6 index cards, and insert them in an inexpensive photo album. Multiples of this gift is easy: just print more copies of each recipe.

To be more creative, consider a theme. Family Favorites, Crock-Pot Time-Savers, or Chocolate Decadence card sets have gift appeal--and next year, add another "set" to the recipient's collection!

Stationery/Label Sets

Practical, consumable, and welcome by everyone from children to young adults to seniors: a packet of computer-printed letterhead and sheets of address labels make a quick, personal gift.

Be creative with graphics, colors and fonts to make this gift more personal and more fun. Put a child's name atop neon-colored paper for a cheerful child's set; give young adults a flashy side border, or embellish a grandmother's stationery with a pretty floral graphic on pastel paper.

Repeat the theme, colors, fonts or graphics on sheets of personalized return address labels, and you've created a perfect, last minute gift.

Bonus: most office supply stores sell matching envelopes for colored papers. Add an envelope set and book of stamps for a more substantial gift.

Gift Coupons

A few minutes work with a word processor and a dash of creativity creates fun "gift coupons". Give children a Cookie-of-the-Month Club certificate good for monthly cookie baking; offer babysitting coupons to parents of young children, or gift older family members with coupons for yard work, repair services, or dinner preparations. Of course, coupons that can be redeemed in hugs and kisses make a fun gift for close family members. Even spicier, give a special spouse coupons for back rubs, bubble baths, or, well, use your imagination!

Cut coupons apart, stack them up, and add a cardstock or construction paper "cover" to the top and bottom. A few staples on the side, and your gift of love is complete.

And Last But Not Least

Christmas Dough Art (Microwave)

4 c all-purpose flour
1 c salt
1 1/2 c hot water*
*Instant coffee added to water gives dough "browned" color.

Knead dough 6 - 8 minutes. Roll out dough and cut with cookie cutters into desired shapes. Place on wax paper on glass tray; with a toothpick, make several holes in each piece to let air escape, then microwave on high for about 2 minutes. Time will vary according to size of "cookies."

INDEX

174

W

Z